T0328533

Understanding Obesity

Most people have some dissatisfaction or concern about body weight, fatness, or obesity, either personally or professionally. This book shows how the popular understanding of obesity is often at odds with scientific understanding, and how misunderstandings about people with obesity can further contribute to the problem. It describes, in an approachable way, interconnected debates about obesity in public policy, medicine and public health, and how media and social media engage people in everyday life in those debates. In chapters considering body fat and fatness, genetics, metabolism, food and eating, inequality, blame and stigma, and physical activity, this book brings separate domains of obesity research into the field of complexity. By doing so, it aids navigation through the minefield of misunderstandings about body weight, fatness and obesity that exist today, after decades of mostly failed policies and interventions.

Stanley Ulijaszek is an anthropologist studying obesity from evolutionary and cultural perspectives. He has undertaken research internationally, in both the Global North and South. He is Director of the Unit for Biocultural Variation and Obesity (UBVO), University of Oxford, which focuses on cultural and policy aspects of body fatness and obesity.

The **Understanding Life** series is for anyone wanting an engaging and concise way into a key biological topic. Offering a multidisciplinary perspective, these accessible guides address common misconceptions and misunderstandings in a thoughtful way to help stimulate debate and encourage a more in-depth understanding. Written by leading thinkers in each field, these books are for anyone wanting an expert overview that will enable clearer thinking on each topic.

Series Editor: Kostas Kampourakis http://kampourakis.com

Published titles:

Understanding Evolution	Kostas Kampourakis	9781108746083
Understanding Coronavirus	Raul Rabadan	9781108826716
Understanding Development	Alessandro Minelli	9781108799232
Understanding Evo-Devo	Wallace Arthur	9781108819466
Understanding Genes	Kostas Kampourakis	9781108812825
Understanding DNA Ancestry	Sheldon Krimsky	9781108816038
Understanding Intelligence	Ken Richardson	9781108940368
Understanding Metaphors in the Life Sciences	Andrew S. Reynolds	9781108940498
Understanding Cancer	Robin Hesketh	9781009005999
Understanding How Science Explains the World	Kevin McCain	9781108995504
Understanding Race	Rob DeSalle and Ian Tattersall	9781009055581
Understanding Human Evolution	Ian Tattersall	9781009101998
Understanding Human Metabolism	Keith N. Frayn	9781009108522
Understanding Fertility	Gab Kovacs	9781009054164
Understanding Forensic DNA	Suzanne Bell and John M. Butler	9781009044011
Understanding Natural Selection	Michael Ruse	9781009088329
Understanding Life in the Universe	Wallace Arthur	9781009207324
Understanding Species	John S. Wilkins	9781108987196

Understanding Obesity

STANLEY ULIJASZEK
University of Oxford

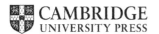

CAMBRIDGE
UNIVERSITY PRESS

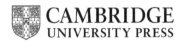
CAMBRIDGE
UNIVERSITY PRESS

Shaftesbury Road, Cambridge CB2 8EA, United Kingdom

One Liberty Plaza, 20th Floor, New York, NY 10006, USA

477 Williamstown Road, Port Melbourne, VIC 3207, Australia

314–321, 3rd Floor, Plot 3, Splendor Forum, Jasola District Centre,
New Delhi – 110025, India

103 Penang Road, #05–06/07, Visioncrest Commercial, Singapore 238467

Cambridge University Press is part of Cambridge University Press & Assessment,
a department of the University of Cambridge.

We share the University's mission to contribute to society through the pursuit of
education, learning and research at the highest international levels of excellence.

www.cambridge.org
Information on this title: www.cambridge.org/9781009218214

DOI: 10.1017/9781009218184

First published 2024

A catalogue record for this publication is available from the British Library

*A Cataloging-in-Publication data record for this book is available from the Library
of Congress*

ISBN 978-1-009-21821-4 Paperback

'This excellent, highly accessible book is for anyone who struggles to make sense of the conflicting portrayals of obesity in our media and across society. Stanley Ulijaszek takes the reader on a fascinating journey from genetics to ultra-processed foods, from swimming to stigma. He explores the latest science to unpick assumptions and misconceptions about obesity in ways that are both enlightening and entertaining, throwing fresh light on this highly complex challenge.'

Harry Rutter, Professor of Global Public Health, University of Bath

'This is a gem! In particular for someone entering obesity research with a wish of acquiring a broader perspective of a complex area. Professor Ulijaszek's profound knowledge, ranging from social, anthropological to biological aspects of obesity is generously shared. He provides the reader with the key steps on how the concepts of obesity have developed historically and how this impacts on the human being today. The writing is crisp and clear, simply a delight to read.'

Fredrik Karpe, Professor of Metabolic Medicine, University of Oxford

'The rising rate of obesity despite scientific and medical advances and dissemination thereof is a complicated paradox – one that warrants careful, thoughtful assessment. Stanley Ulijaszek has furnished just such an assessment in this highly engaging and accessible book, which deftly dissects prominent narrative axioms of the public discourse of obesity and clarifies, in each case, the particular disconnects between science and popular understanding. It's long been clear that obesity is not simply a matter of biology, nor its redress one of the right practice or policy. Accordingly, this careful parsing is a valuable and vital contribution to understanding the myriad contexts and entanglements that shape public understandings of obesity, as well as what productive responses might look like in that complicated terrain.'

Helene A. Shugart, Distinguished Professor of Communication, University of Utah

'Obesity is a complex problem, but in this handy book, Professor Stanley Ulijaszek masterfully explains and simplifies all of the nuances from causes to effects to solutions. With the unique perspective of an anthropologist focussed on food and behaviour, he is able to carefully explain in real simple language why the answer to many of the recurrent questions is "Yes and No". Things aren't always as straightforward as they seem but here we have easy-to-understand explanations of all the important aspects in the obesity equation, from genes to brains, the bugs in your gut, the place where you live, the food we eat and how it's designed and marketed by food companies.'

Michael I. Goran PhD, Professor of Pediatrics and Vice Chair
for Research, Children's Hospital Los Angeles and Keck School
of Medicine at the University of Southern California, and author
of *Sugarproof*

'*Understanding Obesity* reflects on all aspects of obesity, from the more individual to the more societal: genetics, epigenetics, metabolism, stigma, the food environment, food companies, health inequalities and insecurity … Written in a clear and engaging style, it provides an account of the complexity of obesity, calling for multifaceted, carefully considered responses, and inviting us – ultimately – to be more compassionate human beings towards one another. This book could only have been written by someone such as Stanley Ulijaszek who has immense interdisciplinary expertise, an inquisitive mind and a genuine worldwide view. A small but mighty book!'

Amandine Garde, Professor of Law, University of Liverpool

Contents

Foreword

Food has become a central aspect of our lives; not only because we need it in order to live, but also because it has acquired a central part in our socializing – from family gatherings to going out with friends. I recall reading somewhere about a person's concerns with food: 'I spent all day thinking about my next meal and about how to lose weight.' A nice meal offers enjoyment, even more if it is shared with good company. But as Stanley Ulijaszek explains in the present book, in today's societies where food is plentiful, eating for pleasure can result in obesity. And this can be a big problem for at least two reasons: health problems and public shaming. This is then when we begin to ask ourselves: 'Am I too fat?'; 'Is it due to my genes?'; 'Is it due to my metabolism?'; 'Are food corporations or society to blame?'; 'Should I blame myself?'; 'Should I eat less?'; 'Should I go out more?' Ulijaszek considers all these questions one after the other. The result is a marvellous book that addresses widespread misunderstandings about obesity. Things are more complicated than we would like them to be, and therefore the answers and the potential solutions to our concerns are far from simple. What we can do is to begin to realize what the problem really is, and what are its multiple causes. Only then will we be able to deal effectively with it. It is not only about what you can and cannot control. It is not only about you or only about society. It is not only about overeating, and it is not only about exercise. Reading this book will make you see obesity in a new light and reconsider your views about it.

Kostas Kampourakis, Series Editor

Preface

Obesity is one of those confusing issues where everyone has an opinion, and where everyone is invested in their own opinion being right. Why? Because there are few things as personal as your own body, and most people in wealthy societies are unhappy or dissatisfied with theirs in some way. Often this is in relation to body weight and/or fatness. The rich and famous are not exempt in this regard. One day Elon Musk will be part of history, but right now he medicates himself toward a fit body (along with some dietary help and working out) with the latest anti-obesity drug. Even though it is now possible, within constraints, to take a regular jab to reduce body fatness, that is not the end of the story. Silver bullet/single response solutions usually only work for simple problems. They can work for complicated problems too, but they can leave a trail of social and political consequences, as with the emergence of vocal anti-vaxxers in the shadow of the COVID-19 vaccine roll-out. Obesity is neither simple nor complicated. It is complex, involving the interaction of large numbers of factors operating in the evolutionary, historical, and recent past through to the present day, creating predispositions to it, and expression and emergence of it, in response to multiple triggers in social and physical environments now. This book needs to exist, to inform in an approachable way the debate about obesity in policy, medicine, public health and everyday life, because body fatness will continue to roll as a story, a concern and an issue, if only because of the complex nature of its production and the fact that most people have some concern about their body.

From the start of my engagement with obesity as something to research and understand, back in the 1990s, my focus has been of the non-medical type.

Concentrating on social and societal aspects of body fatness, as befits an anthropologist, has allowed me to study relationships of obesity with politics and economics, metrics of the body and of the body in society, of food and eating, of urbanism and of physical activity. With extraordinarily talented colleagues, I have investigated how obesity is related to social and physical environments, to inequality, insecurity, neoliberalism, colonialism, and stigma, forming the imperfect storm, made up differently in different contexts, that has proven impossible to calm, even with all the promises that have been made to 'conquer' obesity across the decades.

The issues associated with obesity are interconnected and entangled. The chapters of this book offer understandings located in evolution and biology, but also society and politics, as well as complexity. Each chapter pulls on one or several of the entangled threads that constitute obesity as an issue, shedding light, busting myths, and clearing up some of the many misunderstandings about it. The words 'obesity', 'fatness' and 'weight' are used to give discursive substance to three overlapping but slightly differing ideas. Body weight is just that – the sum total, in pounds or kilograms, of what someone weighs. When I put on or take off body weight (as an adult) I use body weight as a proxy for gaining or losing body fatness. This is a working approximation, since for most people weight change is largely due to change in fat mass (but not always – it can also be due to whether they are hydrated or not, working out and gaining muscle, or bed-ridden with illness and losing muscle). Body fat is one constituent of body weight (in addition to muscle, bone, extra-cellular fluid) and is distributed across the body within cells of the adipose tissue.

Body fat is demonized by many in an indiscriminate way, but actually, much body fat and adipose tissue (according to its location) does useful and life-enhancing things. Obesity is body fatness excessive relative to norms, to an extent that it is associated with disease and death. The term 'obesity' is a medical one and has been contested by people who disagree with the label because they disagree with bodies (their own and of others) being subjected to norms, and because the label itself is stigmatizing. Much more is said about this in Chapter 1. Genetic associations with obesity and body fatness are plentiful but difficult to comprehend in an easy manner, and this is the subject of Chapter 2. Obesity may never have existed in previous human evolutionary history except in individuals with comparatively rare genetics – so-called monogenic obesity. In the present day, people with monogenic obesity represent a very small proportion of all people with obesity, the vast majority developing a so-called 'common' form involving many genes and gene regions. There are several ways of understanding obesity from evolutionary and genetic perspectives, and these are also discussed in this chapter. Chapter 3 considers the mechanisms of energy metabolism as they relate to obesity, engaging with the physiology of body fat deposition, genetics, and neurobiology of appetite. Chapter 4 goes on to consider obesity in relation to the food environment, focusing on systems of food production and distribution that have led to the widespread availability of cheap ultra-processed foods (UPFs). What follows in Chapter 5 is an examination of how social processes influence obesity rates. Stress and inequalities in income and education play their part, as does the insecurity that comes with living in a neoliberal society. Still in the social domain, Chapter 6 unpacks how body stigma works, and how it contributes to obesity, and how in turn, obesity contributes to stigma. It considers the moralizing background that underpins this nasty social evaluative practice, and how this practice is used to maintain social hierarchy in societies where there is plentiful food. In Chapter 7, reasons why it is difficult for many people to regulate their appetites are given and expanded upon. Some people can very easily overeat without noticeable effect, while others just need to sniff a doughnut (metaphorically speaking) to gain weight. There is a mismatch between our fundamental biology, which has evolved to want to eat and find satisfaction in calories, and food production systems that provide calories easily and cheaply. The question of why UPFs are liked so much is considered, as well as the question of how not all dietary calories are equal. Chapter 8 examines physical activity in relation to body weight, and the physical location of adipose tissue in and on the body. Chapter 9 considers how the many factors associated with obesity combine in a cocktail of complexity, which varies in composition for different populations and countries across time. While complexity is where obesity research has travelled to, media messaging about body fatness and obesity has hardly changed across decades, making it difficult to disseminate the most current knowledge about obesity to broader audiences. The logic of media representation of obesity is thus also considered in this chapter.

Throughout the book, there is commentary about what can be done at population level in governance and policy, and by individuals, and through personal agency, to come to terms with obesity, body fatness and body weight. Where in the text I give brief snatches of conversations with people, the names are fictionalized, but the paraphrased conversations are real, unless I state otherwise. I hope you find the book as interesting to read as it has been to write. Above all I hope you find it useful in helping you to structure how you think about this complex topic. For anyone interested in following up on anything, my email address is stanley.ulijaszek@anthro.ox.ac.uk.

Acknowledgements

I especially thank younger colleagues with whom I have worked on obesity and related matters for their honest and generous critique of various chapters. Your input has strengthened this work. A big thank you goes to each of – Amy McLennan, of the Australian National University; Helene Shugart, of the University of Utah; Michelle Pentecost, of King's College London; Tanja Schneider, of the University of St Gallen; Karin Eli; Zofia Boni, of the Adam Mickiewicz University, Poznan; Tess Bird and Sabine Parrish, both of the University of Oxford; Anne Katrine Kleberg Hansen, of the Royal Danish Academy of Arts, Copenhagen; Thao Dam, of Maastricht University; and Esther Gonzalez-Padilla, of Lund University.

I thank Caroline Potter, of the University of Oxford, for her continued involvement in the Unit for BioCultural Variation and Obesity (UBVO – www.oxfordobesity .org) at the University of Oxford, most recently as Co-Director, with myself and Karin Eli, of the University of Warwick. This interdisciplinary network of researchers was formed in 2007, and I thank Devi Sridhar, of the University of Edinburgh, for her involvement at its inception.

I thank the Magic Table, a group of scholars and writers who share and critique each other's writing in very kind and constructive ways. I am very privileged to be part of it. Members of the Magic Table are acknowledged by name above – you know who you are.

It is wonderful that my editors, Kostas Kampourakis and Jessica Papworth, are invested in making this the best of all possible popular books on obesity. Thank you, Kostas, for your generous critique of the entire book.

I thank many of the great and the good in obesity science and beyond, that I have had the privilege of meeting and knowing, for great discussions and conversations about the body, fatness, and obesity. Thanks to all – Giles Yeo, Amandine Garde, William Dietz, Rebecca Puhl, Karen Throsby, Bethan Evans, Marion Nestle, Jane Wardle, Robert Fogel, Adam Drewnowski, Gema Frubeck, John Komlos, Rachel Colls, Megan Warin, Maciej Henneberg, Michael Davies, Vivienne Moore, Cat Pause, Thorkild Sorensen, Erik Hemmingsson, Line Hillesdal, Paulina Nowicka, Claude Marcus, Finn Rasmussen, Lena Hansson, Fredrik Karpe, David Hull, Michael Stock, Dame Nancy Rothwell, Hannah Graff, Sir Michael Marmot, Jonathan Wells, Tim Lobstein, Philip James, Anna Lavis, Emma Jayne Abbots, Anna Carden-Coyne, Kelvin Chan, James Stubbs, Catriona Bonfiglioli, Geof Rayner, Boyd Swinburn, Bruno Latour, Michael Goran, Emily Henderson, Heather Howard, Osea Giuntella, Dan Nettle, Lord Sir John Krebs, Robin Dunbar, Mike Rayner, Cecilia Lindgren, Danny Dorling, Hayley Lofink, Avner Offer, Susan Jebb, Keith Frayn, Jimmy Bell, Jennifer Baker, Nic Timpson, George Davey Smith, Kate Pickett, Richard Wilkinson, Chris Forth, Michael Goran, Michel Belot, Franco Sassi, Shirlene Badger, Mel Wenger, Vivienne Parry, Rosie Kay, Oli Williams, Emma Rich, Harry Rutter, Susan Greenhalgh. To anyone I may have omitted, I give my deep apologies.

I thank Fellows and students of the very wonderful St Cross College Oxford, for stimulating discussions, usually over lunch, about obesity, body fatness and the body, and many more things besides – how to think about complexity, globalization, insecurity, for example. Things that relate to obesity, and much, much more.

I thank members of the very inclusive and extensive open water swimming community in the United Kingdom and beyond, especially members of the Serpentine Swimming Club, London, and fellow swimmers in Oxford and Oxfordshire, for their camaraderie, bonhomie, and year-round immersion in the blue outdoors. Many water-side discussions (often over a hot drink) on many of the issues presented in this book, with interested non-specialists (mostly swimmers), have helped me present this work in an accessible style.

Above all I thank my immediate family – Pauline, Michael, Alexandra, Peter – for their interest as I have been writing this book into existence, and in keeping me grounded.

1 I'm Too Fat

Hot Potato

I have met few adults who are happy with their own bodies, at least in Western societies. But even in non-Western societies, many people are unhappy with their bodies. The exact nature of this unhappiness varies, but what overwhelmingly dominates is the thought, whether objectively true or not, that they carry too much weight, and following that, the thought that they really should lose weight. I have met very few people who actively want to put on weight, and they have almost all been of athletic disposition, and the weight gain sought is usually (but not always) in terms of muscle. Some people are entirely 'fat-phobic' and not persuaded that some types of body fat might actually be good, healthy even. Many people don't know that there are different types of fat deposit, and that some deposits of fatness carry limited or no negative health consequences – around the buttocks, hips and thighs, for example. Body fatness is a 'hot potato' issue for many people; I like hot potatoes.

But what is excess or pathological body fatness? How would you define it, beyond 'I know it when I see it'? And what are the different types of body fat? And does the fat I eat become the fat on my body? This book is for all the people who worry about their weight and/or their body fatness, which is to say, most people. Body fatness, good fat, bad fat, what I call ugly fat, the imperfect science of how fatness relates to illness, how obesity is measured, and how and why people judge people who carry extra weight – all of these things are considered.

The different types of body fat evolved along with the rest of our bodies. For our ancestors, consuming energy-dense foods and conserving dietary energy through gaining weight and as body fat could have provided a reproductive advantage then, if no longer in the present day. Such potentially evolved tendencies and mechanisms towards positive energy balance and weight gain are complex, and complexity is my lens for viewing obesity, through approaches as diverse as evolutionary theory, physiology, neurobiology, sociology and anthropology.

How did I get interested in obesity as a subject of research? I am an anthropologist, not a public health specialist, nor a medic. I am interested in people and communities, less so in risk groups, and even less so in disease and disability, except in as far as they impact on personal and social lives. Obesity is far more complex than being a disease related to body fatness, as some have framed it. It is something that can socially divide people, bringing out the worst in some, with stigmatization and shaming of people carrying excess body fatness. If it is a disease (which many experts and health agencies think it is), it is as much a social disease (in terms of fat phobia and stigmatization) as a medical one. I became interested in body fatness and obesity because my anthropological fieldwork in Papua New Guinea (PNG) into traditional subsistence and nutritional ecology (that is, how people's nutritional needs are attained in the environment in which they live) took me there. I first went to the Purari Delta region of the country in the late 1970s, when undernutrition and infection were the big health-related issues. I felt I had understood and defined the problem quite well by the time I left some two years later, well enough to help define policies and interventions, to make a difference. When I went back to this rural area 14 years later, my pleasure in seeing the great reduction in undernutrition was cancelled out by seeing many people with overnutrition and obesity, which had previously been nonexistent. I couldn't fathom how this could have happened in less than a generation. In the mid-1990s I switched focus to obesity, not because of the emergent public health problem associated with it, but because of this swift and dramatic shift in nutritional health in a group of people I had worked with in remote PNG. It didn't fit the dominant narrative of the time, which was of obesity as a problem predominating in the Global North. I am always attracted by an anomaly.

Subsequent fieldwork in the Cook Islands, and analysis of inequality and obesity data from socialist and post-socialist Poland, both got me thinking and researching the different ways in which obesity seemed to manifest itself in different populations. By the mid-2000s, over a hundred factors associated with obesity had been identified by researchers across the field of study, and it was time for a new approach, harnessing interaction and layering, which led me, via obesity policy think-tank work, to complexity, and setting up the Unit for BioCultural Variation and Obesity (UBVO) in 2007 at the University of Oxford. The work of this group has since informed obesity policy at the World Health Organization (WHO), and the governments of the United Kingdom (UK), Denmark, and Sweden.

This book is very much guided by the framings used by UBVO, using ecological, anthropological, social and political approaches to body fatness and obesity, and placing them within a biocultural context. In biocultural anthropology, the relationships between human biology and culture are paramount. With a biocultural approach to obesity, it is the anthropology of body fatness that is in the spotlight – its social, cultural, evolutionary, environmental aspects, rather than its medical and public health framings, although biocultural approaches do inform medicine and public health.

The easy narrative attached to obesity, which is that if you eat too much and don't get enough exercise you will put on body fat, isn't helpful for understanding different patterns of obesity increase across the world, Global North and Global South. Across decades of research into obesity, in Australia, India, Denmark, Sweden, Poland, the United States (US) and the UK, I have tripped over many misunderstandings. My hope is that this book will help you walk through the minefield of misunderstanding with more confidence. I can't guarantee that you won't stumble – there are probably still many unexploded misunderstandings about obesity – but hopefully this book can help guide you through.

Body Fat – What Is the Good of It?

In nature, body fatness is usually a good thing. As a species, humans have greater capability of accumulating body fat than non-human primates. Placing this in evolutionary context reveals the adaptive value of body fatness.

The rapid brain evolution that came with the emergence of our *Homo erectus* ancestor almost 2 million years ago was probably associated with increased body fatness as well as diet quality – the greater availability of dietary animal fat and cholesterol is likely to have allowed encephalization, or increased brain size relative to the size of the body. Higher levels of body fatness and lower muscle mass relative to other primate species have allowed human infants to accommodate brain growth by having adequate stored energy for brain metabolism. Since energy stores are vital to survivorship and reproduction, the ability to conserve energy as adipose tissue would have conferred selective advantage in the food-constrained environments that early *Homo sapiens* would have been periodically exposed to. Fatness was crucial to the reproduction of ancestral humans and continues to be so in contemporary society. In females it is linked to fertility, and ovarian function is sensitive to energy balance and energy flux. At any body mass index (BMI), females have a greater proportion of their body weight as fat than males. Furthermore, they have a greater proportion of their fat in the lower body than do males, fat which is mobilized during pregnancy and lactation.

These very successful adaptations – in energy metabolism, in fat storage – have become burdens in the present day, as global food security issues were conquered in the 50 years or so since the 1960s, at least in relation to production of dietary energy. This was a period when the world's then-dominant nutritional problem, that of undernutrition, could have been fixed, but instead, a steady decline in people suffering undernutrition was to some extent matched by rising obesity. There are many places in the present day where an individual might even experience both undernutrition (especially in early childhood) and overnutrition (in adult life). More about this in Chapter 2. This rise in obesity is undoubtedly due to a wide range of associated and interrelated factors, with the inundation of the global food market with cheap calories (a triumph of industrial agriculture if you will) having underwritten it.

What Is Obesity and How Is It Measured?

Obesity (as defined by contemporary measures of the body mass index, or BMI) was retrospectively identified by economic historian John Komlos, of the University of Munich, as an emergent population phenomenon among North

American men in the nineteenth century. Obesity then rose across the twentieth century, accelerating with the rise of global capitalism and neoliberalism from the 1980s onwards. It became a matter of economic concern in the US and the UK in the 1990s, when its direct health costs became clear. Economics, medicine and public health have framed obesity as particular types of problem to be controlled or managed in some way. However, it is not a problem for everyone. Nor is it the same problem for everyone concerned about obesity. So, for whom is obesity a problem, and why?

This was a question we posed in the very first seminar series of UBVO. Researchers interested in obesity as an object of research have different ways of thinking about it, which is only natural given that researchers will engage with a problem with their best theory, not someone else's – they can only do what they have trained to do. What is interesting is how differently different disciplines frame obesity and excess body fatness. For political scientists, obesity is a problem of governance, while for epidemiologists it is one of accelerating mortality and morbidity. For some economists, it is an unintended consequence of some types of economic system; for food systems analysts, a problem of incomplete specification. There were many approaches taken by researchers presenting at this first UBVO seminar series, confirming obesity to be a subject that requires interdisciplinary approaches. For people with obesity, there are other considerations, like stigma, blame and occupational glass ceilings. For many young adults with obesity who do not suffer the chronic disease consequences of it, it may not be seen as a problem at all. What appears to be commonly accepted is an evolutionary basis to body fatness, which is where I turn next, followed by a discussion of how excess body weight is defined.

You can go far in understanding obesity without defining it, and its definition has in recent decades been linked to understanding it as a disease state (or not), associated with mortality (or not). In 2014, the WHO defined obesity as 'abnormal or excessive fat accumulation that may impair health'. What exactly 'abnormal' or 'excessive' levels of body fatness are in relation to health continue to be debated among obesity researchers. There are some clear answers to these questions, but only at the extremes of body weight and fatness. This is good enough for medics to act – with obesity surgery at the high extreme of body fatness, and treatment for anorexia nervosa at the low – but for public health, mild or moderate obesity is coloured in shades of grey. At what point should any professional body or institution intervene? There is no clear and unambiguous answer. For the social scientist, how medics deal with severe obesity is a subject of study in its own right, as is how public health authorities define and act on less extreme forms of body fatness. The study of bodily norms and how they are socially enforced, and understandings of what constitutes health for any individual or group, are subjects of investigation for anthropologists. With many different stakeholders and approaches, it is easy to see what a fraught matter obesity has become.

The question 'Is obesity a disease?' has never been fully answered. Many agencies, governmental and other, view it as such, with the WHO and the US National Institutes of Health having done so from the 1990s. Jantina de Vries, then of the University of Oxford, argued in 2007 against classifying it as a disease. From an evolutionary perspective, she asserted that if some bodily conditions either confer evolutionary or biological advantage or are common to a species, they should not be regarded as diseases; only if bodily conditions are rare and fall out of the range of morphological normality should they be considered thus. Body fatness is typical of the human species, and on this basis, obesity cannot be considered to be a disease. From a societal perspective, she argued that obesity can be framed as disease because it represents bodily deviation from norms and social desirability. George Bray, then of the Pennington Biomedical Research Center at Louisiana State University, argued in the early 2000s that obesity is a chronic relapsing neurological disease, requiring lifelong treatment or management. Lifelong intervention means lifelong employment for those involved in its treatment, as well as the growth of an industry built around anti-obesity interventions, which in the US in 2022 alone was worth nearly 150 billion dollars.

Whether disease or not, there is a judgement call on how excess body fatness should be measured – there are lots of ways of doing it – and it matters, at least for the obesity treatment and management industry. If you don't have a consensus on defining obesity, you can't really intervene.

So how is it measured? The simplest measure out there is body weight – you just stand on the scale and judge for yourself according to what you think you should weigh. You might want to relate that to norms of body weight, or weight for height, or weight over height squared (the BMI). I personally ignore the BMI when considering my own body weight. For the record, my BMI tips into the overweight category but only just. I don't agonize over it, but monitor my weight, trying to neither lose nor gain it. I know how much attention and discipline is needed to lose weight, and I want to avoid the stress of constant vigilance over what I eat. If you want to measure excess body fatness or obesity by BMI, for medical or public health intervention for example, then norms become more important. Weight alone doesn't take into account differences in height between people; if you are taller, you are likely to be heavier, just because you are carrying a bigger skeleton – a bigger frame on which to pack both muscle and fat. One measure of obesity that makes allowance for this is weight for height. This doesn't entirely neutralize differences in weight due to differences in height, however. The BMI – weight (in kilograms) divided by the square of height (in metres) – does a better job in neutralizing the effects of height on weight, but does so in a far from perfect way.

The BMI was formalized for international use by the WHO in 2000, with several aims: to make the assessment and monitoring of obesity worldwide as simple as possible; to allow public health authorities to make meaningful comparisons within and between populations; to identify individuals and groups at increased risk of disease and death; to help identify priorities for intervention at individual and community levels; and to give a basis for evaluating interventions. For epidemiological investigation, this formalization rendered meaningless population estimates of obesity based on measures other than BMI, or that used different norms or cut-offs for obesity. In epidemiology, the BMI is used as a proxy for body energy stores, and at the upper end of a population distribution it shows strong but imperfect associations with a number of chronic diseases and disorders, both in morbidity and mortality. Other measures such as waist circumference, waist to hip ratio, and waist to height ratio compete very well with it, so it is worth considering why the BMI continues to be a standard measure of obesity.

The BMI works just about well enough for epidemiological and public health work. It has been used for far longer than any other anthropometric measure and was the first to be appropriated for the assessment of obesity rates in populations. It is collected systematically across the world – no other measure is, to anywhere near the same extent. One reason for this is that heights and weights are relatively easy to measure. Just over a decade ago, the WHO considered switching to one of a small number of measures that incorporate waist circumference, but decided against it. This is because changing the standard measure of global obesity surveillance would have thrown the international governance of obesity into disarray, at a time when obesity was rising fast (it continues to rise). Obesity measurement and reporting allows the tracking of obesity across time and in different countries, giving background data for anti-obesity interventions. In most countries, obesity is reported in terms of the proportion of adults with a BMI greater than 30 kg/m^2, although lower cut-offs are deemed appropriate for people of Asian ancestry, whose disease and death risk is higher at any BMI point than for people of European ancestry. For people of Pacific Islander ancestry, higher cut-offs are deemed appropriate, because such populations carry lower disease and death risk at any BMI point.

The BMI measure does a lot of work for public health obesity, but does it do as much for you and me as individuals? Well, it depends. While BMI cut-offs for obesity classification are seen as meaningful for epidemiological and public health work, health and well-being can be perceived quite differently by people who have been classified as having obesity. For example, Helen Doll, and her colleagues at the University of Oxford, have shown that the self-reported health status of adults in the UK is low among people categorized as having severe obesity, with BMI greater than 40 (Figure 1.1), but lowest among people with any category of obesity also experiencing chronic disease (Figure 1.2). Thus, obesity may not be a problem for people with non-severe obesity if they do not also experience chronic illness.

Two criticisms of BMI are that it's not just the amount of fat that you carry that's important, but where you carry it, and that it can only give an imperfect measure of overall body fatness at the individual level. Fat on the thighs and bum protects against chronic disease, while fat in the abdomen harms. Among physically fit people, high BMI can reflect muscularity more than fatness. Natalie King, of the University of Leeds, and her colleagues did a study of body composition of players in the four teams taking part in the semi-finals of the 2003 Rugby Union World Cup. Nine out of ten of them had a BMI that would categorize them as either overweight or obese by the WHO criteria, when in fact they were extremely muscular, and the BMI picked that up.

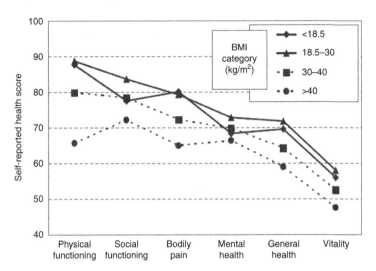

Figure 1.1   Distribution of self-reported health scores by body mass index (BMI) category, after adjusting for age, gender and frequency of health service utilization, in the UK.

Jimmy Bell, of Imperial College London, has perfected techniques for whole body imaging of human body fat distribution. He found that there are people with high BMI who, because of their fat distribution, do not carry a health risk equivalent to their upper-range BMI. As a result, he came up with the acronym TOFI – thin on the outside, fat on the inside. A person he might identify as TOFI would have a BMI in the normal range but carry fat in their abdomen, carrying a health risk as a consequence. Between 10 and 30 per cent of people classified as having obesity by the BMI classification have metabolically healthy obesity (MHO). There is no standardized definition of MHO, but all start with obesity as defined by BMI $\geq$ 30 kg/m^2, in combination with one or more of the following markers that are associated with health rather than chronic disease: low fasted serum triglycerides; elevated HDL cholesterol serum concentrations; systolic and diastolic blood pressures in the normative range; low fasting blood glucose; an absence of drug treatment for dyslipidae-mia, diabetes or hypertension; and no cardiovascular disease manifestations.

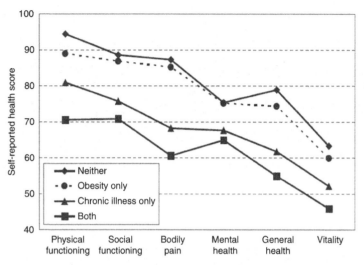

Figure 1.2   Distribution of self-reported health scores (the higher the healthier) according to obesity (defined by BMI) and chronic illness, after adjusting for age, gender and frequency of health service utilization, in the UK.

Clinical scientists remain cautious about calling MHO truly healthy until there is clear evidence across a number of years to that effect.

But there is clear evidence that the BMI does not distinguish between different types of body fat and their locations. This is an important consideration for thinking about obesity in relation to disease, which is what the next section examines.

Is Some Fat OK?

The BMI is not able to distinguish between potentially harmful fat in the liver and abdomen (around the viscera) and less harmful fat under the skin, in the buttocks or thighs. Fat accumulated in the abdomen and liver has been linked epidemiologically to cardiovascular disease, type 2 diabetes and death due to all causes, while fat beneath the skin, especially in the lower body, is neutral, or even protective against chronic disease. Visceral fat is more easily mobilized by physical activity than is subcutaneous fat, and a high BMI is of much less concern if you are physically active and carry a lot of muscle. The all-cause and cardiovascular (CVD) risk of death in people with obesity who are physically fit (on the basis of cardiorespiratory fitness) is no different to people in the normal range of BMI who are also fit (that is, the theoretically healthiest group). Where your fat is deposited matters, for health.

In the Italian language, good is good, and bad can be ugly, or not. Which is to say that ugly can also mean bad, depending on context – 'ugly' is thus a moral category as well as an aesthetic one. Taking this to body fatness, fat can be good, bad, or morally ugly.

We all carry fat on and in our bodies, and in general, this is a good thing. It is an evolved bodily characteristic and has many benefits. We carry it in the form of triglycerides in adipose tissue, and adipose tissue does many useful things to help keep us alive. For starters, adipose tissue is an insulator, protecting our bodies against the cold. Subcutaneous adipose tissue acts as a biological overcoat. Some animal species that haven't got much body fat have body fur. Across evolutionary time we have lost our ability to grow fur and gained the ability to develop body fatness – in fact, we are the fattest of all primate species. Humans do a lot both behaviourally and culturally (if we call technology a part of culture) to keep ourselves warm and to avoid having to call upon our body fat as an insulator – what with clothing, housing, central heating, heating in cars, bedding, and so on. We can survive a moderate amount of cold exposure, but shivering usually kicks in before we get too cold, to defend our core body temperature.

Adipose tissue is a good energy store, fat offering nine calories of energy per gram that can be used in metabolism, compared with four for each of carbohydrate and protein respectively. Being able to store energy as fat contributed to our evolutionary success as a species. Seasonality in temperature and periodic food shortage were major environmental pressures in human evolution, and being able to store energy as fat on the body was an important adaptation. It continues to be important for people living in seasonal environments in the rural Global South now. It is also important for women having babies, both past and in the present day, where body fat gained in pregnancy contributes energy for breast milk production, one of the most physiologically costly things for a woman.

Adipose tissue is also involved in innate and adaptive immunity, the day-to-day protection against disease we usually take for granted. It makes and stores a range of immune system proteins that identify disease-causing bacteria, viruses and fungi and help neutralize them before they can do any damage to our bodies. A number of proteins made and stored in the adipose tissue have dual purpose – to act immunologically, protecting against disease, but also in metabolism, most importantly mediating the work of insulin, the powerful body cell-building and bodily maintenance hormone. Adipose tissue also makes and secretes hormones that help to regulate appetite, energy balance and reproduction. According to Miguel Otero of Santiago University, Spain, and his colleagues, the hormone leptin, produced in adipose tissue, is a critical link between adipose tissue, the regulation of appetite by the brain, and energy balance, as well as being important in immunological memory, and in glucorticoid metabolism in mediating the immune response. Leptin is also involved in haematopoiesis (the production of all of the cellular components of blood and blood plasma), in angiogenesis (the formation of new blood vessels), in fetal development and in maturation of the reproductive system.

Adipose tissue – where would we be without it? 'Dead' is the answer to that question. Some specialist forms of adipose tissue can produce heat when we are exposed to cold stress. This is brown adipose tissue, or BAT for short. Masayuki Saito, formerly of Hokkaido University, and colleagues found greater activation of BAT in winter compared with summer in human subjects, as well as BAT activity being inversely related to BMI, and to visceral fat content. They suggested that BAT, because of its energy-dissipating activity, must be protective against body fat accumulation, and therefore also obesity. Different people have different levels of BAT activity, and this was once thought to be why some people can eat plentifully and not put on weight while others can't. Eating induces heat production with diet-induced thermo-genesis (DIT), the energy we use in digesting food, and this too is mediated by BAT. The activation of heat production in BAT by both cold exposure and eating operates through the stimulation of the sympathetic nervous system.

The stimulatory effects of cold exposure on BAT are also mediated through transient receptor potential (TRP) channels, having something in common with the effects of capsaicin consumption – think of eating food spiced with chilli peppers. Most of the different types of TRP channels sense chemical compounds which are ultimately perceived variously as pain, touch or temperature. With food, they can be described as spiciness or pungency, for example, and the perception of a spicy food can vary with the physical temperature of a food. I don't know if it is just me, but when eating cold curry the day after its making, it seems much less spicy than when I ate it hot the evening before. Capsaicin, and some molecules very similar to it, mimic the effects of cold exposure to decrease body fatness through the activation and recruitment of BAT. Green tea may do something similar because of the catechins it contains, but this hasn't yet been fully researched.

We wouldn't be alive without body fat and the adipose tissue it is stored in, so it is a great shame that people often feel very negatively about their own bodily fat. Ugly fat, I call it, the ugliness lying in how it is perceived, and not so much in its healthiness or otherwise. Ugly fat, body fatness associated with aesthetics and perception, how people judge people who carry extra weight (including themselves), is what the popular debate concerning the BMI is mostly about, perhaps more so than about health. Perceptions of appropriate body size for health and beauty vary and change across societies and time (Chapters 5 and 6). Sociocultural factors, including participation in the global economy and exposure to Western ideas and ideals, influence them, there being a general and global trend towards increased valuation of thinness and increased awareness of the health risks of obesity. There are a number of communities and societies where obesity rates have risen in recent decades where previously people preferred or accepted larger body size as attractive, and where they now prefer thinner bodies. These include African Americans, Pacific Islanders, Native Americans and people in South Korea. Among Europeans, the desire for thinness used to be a privilege of wealthier classes since the late nineteenth century, and has become more widespread in the past half century or so. The higher cultural valuation of body fatness has become a thing of the past in most places.

The present-day linking of beauty to the lean and fit body has deep roots in the history of Western thought. The democratic dissemination of this ideal, alongside the new industry of self-improvement and the diet industry, really took off only around four decades ago. The athletic and youthfully packaged fit thin body is what now serves as a marker of social status and cultural capital for women; for men tallness and muscularity suffice. These ideals of beauty linked to fitness are set within neoliberal norms of self-marketing (Chapter 5), where seeing is believing, and where moral judgement of fat bodies is easy, because they are publicly visible, even when covered by clothing. The Italian word 'brutto' is not just visibly ugly but can be morally so. There's an echo of this in the English language – 'as ugly as sin'. Social perceptions, perceptions of others, have a strong influence on self-perception of body fatness. As a result of negative attitudes toward fatness, there is much stigmatization of people carrying excess body fatness, and body image disturbance is common, not just among people classified as having obesity. Individuals with weight within the normal range of its classification often have difficulty in accurately assessing their body size, and who view their own body fatness, even if healthy, as ugly. There is plentiful evidence of stress and stigmatization doing damage to health, independently of body fatness. Add body fatness to the mix, and it is so much worse.

The bad fat in our bodies includes deep subcutaneous adipose tissue (dSAT), visceral fat, and fat in the liver. dSAT was identified by Gillian Walker and her colleagues, at the Italian Institute of Auxology in Piancavallo, Italy, as a distinct form of abdominal adipose tissue which is involved in the development of obesity-associated chronic disease complications including metabolic syndrome (Chapter 3). Visceral fat accumulates around the intestine and is associated with fatty acid profiles in the blood that can lead to cardiovascular disease. Fat infiltrating the liver (hepatic steatosis) is strongly associated with the metabolic syndrome regardless of whether you carry excess fat in the rest of your body or not. If the liver is constantly exposed to free fatty acids (FFA), fat is deposited there, from a failure of being able to oxidize the excess for immediate use as bodily energy. There is a strong association between abdominal obesity, elevated FFA levels and fatty liver, visceral fat being the key driver of fatty liver development. Visceral fat and fatty liver are the key components of obesity-related disease. Having examined the different types of adipose tissue, I next turn to diseases associated with obesity.

Disease Risks

In 2009, the WHO placed obesity among the leading global risks of death. Of the diseases associated with it, type 2 diabetes, cardiovascular diseases, a range of cancers, fatty liver disease, kidney disease and respiratory disease are the most common, both in prevalence of disease and in deaths from them. Death associated with obesity is higher in men than in women, mostly because men are more likely to develop cardiovascular diseases and cancers than are women. This in turn is largely because they are more likely to have practised health-risky behaviour across their lives than women, as well being less likely to seek healthcare or advice when ill. Testosterone also promotes cell growth and therefore the progressive of cancer, whereas oestrogen protects against cardiovascular disease and breast cancer. Obesity is also a major cause of chronic inflammation, especially in later life, this being a common pathway for chronic disease development. The inflammation associated with severe obesity was a major reason why people contracting COVID-19 in the early months of the pandemic were more likely to end up in intensive care than people in the normative range of BMI. I am put in mind of the British Prime Minister of the time, Boris Johnson, who had poo-pooed obesity as an important object for policy, only to change his mind after recovering from near-fatal COVID-19. In recovery, medics informed him that his then BMI of 36 kg/m^2 had almost certainly tipped him to the edge of death.

Even with mass vaccination against COVID-19, obesity continues to be a major factor in the development and severity of this infectious disease. Professor Sir Aziz Sheik of the University of Edinburgh and his colleagues have found that even with COVID-19 vaccination, people with obesity are at higher risk of developing severe infection than people with weight in the normative range, the extent of protection from vaccination dropping off faster for people with severe obesity. There are many other diseases and disorders associated with obesity that are less likely to cause death, but that are worrying and painful nonetheless. These include obstructive sleep apnoea, gallstones, glomerulosclerosis, joint problems, menstrual irregularities, osteoporosis and polycystic ovary syndrome.

Obesity has increased in children and adolescents, and this has increased the risk of chronic disease and death in adult life, partly because of an extended period of life carrying excess weight and consuming diets high in saturated fats and refined carbohydrates, both of which are associated with elevated chronic disease risk independently of obesity. Cardiovascular disease risk is also raised among those at the lower end of the BMI scale in childhood, but who develop excess weight in adulthood. More about this in Chapter 2.

What Can We Do?

There are so many factors associated with obesity that it might seem difficult to know where to start. We can focus on the interactive and complex nature of obesity, of which more in Chapter 9. As individuals, we can be more forgiving of ourselves and of others who might be carrying excess weight, knowing how our physiology has been shaped across evolutionary time to make it easy to put on weight, and so difficult to lose it. More about this in Chapters 3 and 7. We can think about how stigma and blame against people carrying excess weight has become entrenched in wealthy nations, and how we might respond to this within society and as individuals – this is discussed in Chapters 5 and 6.

I have mentioned energy balance a few times in this chapter, but have purposely avoided any suggestion that it is energy imbalance, that is, calories eaten exceeding calories expended by the body in different ways across a prolonged period (usually years), that causes obesity. There will be much more about this in Chapter 3, but there is every possibility that scientists, policymakers, medical practitioners have been barking up the wrong tree for almost half a century, and that focusing on energy imbalance might even have contributed to obesity. It is important to sort out whether calories in total are more important than the type of calories that come into our bodies, because this has profound implications for our food systems and what we individually choose or are able to eat on a daily basis.

We can acknowledge that our genetics contributes to obesity, but that apart from rare types of single-gene forms of obesity, we can't pin it down precisely. More about this in Chapter 2. We can blame the food corporations for selling us poor food and persuading us that it is good. More about this in Chapters 4 and 7. We can look at how we move around in our daily lives, and how the structures of urban places either help or hinder physical activity. More on this in Chapter 8.

Now read on.

2 It's My Genes

Genie in a Bottle

People have asked me if their body fatness is genetic, to which I reply unhelpfully, yes and no. There is a very tiny proportion of any population that very easily puts on weight, where a small number of genes relate to, or are implicated in, excessive weight gain. There is a larger group of people with several genes that are triggered by one or several of a range of environmental factors to gain body fatness. And then there is almost everyone else, each person with thousands of genetic variants that have seemingly small individual effects in relation to obesity under circumstances that favour it. There are also those annoying people who can eat as much as they want, of anything they want, and not put on weight, seemingly with genes for thinness. The study of obesity genetics is steadily letting the genie out of the bottle – once you know something, you can't unknow it, and we know enough about this area now to be able to reply with 'It depends', when someone says, 'My body fatness is down to my genes.'

There are several evolutionary arguments about how genetics and obesity are linked, from the classic 'thrifty gene' hypothesis of the 1960s to the 'drifty gene' hypothesis of the early 2000s, both suggesting alternative ways in which genetic predispositions to obesity might have evolved and how they might operate in the present day. There is also a predator hypothesis of obesity which was framed in the 2000s, in which an ecological basis for the evolution of genes associated with body fatness is proposed. These and other theories of obesity genetics are discussed in this chapter. There is currently no grand narrative of obesity genetics, this being a site still very much under construction.

Without genetic predispositions to obesity there would be no obesity, that's for sure. While it's tempting to say, 'My genes made me do it' – eat too much cake, avoid exercise, stay at home when I should have gone for a walk, reach for the television remote, surf the web and endlessly watch funny memes on social media – I wish it could be that simple. The truth of it is that you might have genetics that increase your likelihood of putting on weight, or make you hungry at the drop of a cheesecake, or make you wear active wear while sitting on the sofa watching YouTube work-out videos, but they don't do their stuff on their own. There needs to be something in the environment that makes the genetics switch on (or off). Like, you might want cheesecake, but if there isn't any, you can't do anything with the craving for it. Or you might not want to get out of bed, but you have to, to get to your place of work on a Monday morning. There are aspects of the built environment that can predispose to obesity, but not everyone is influenced by them in ways that can lead to obesity. Genetics needs environmental triggers to switch on and make it work. This is called gene expression, and there is a huge amount of it going on, all the time, especially in relation to the food you eat. For thousands of years, people have carried copies of common genes that we now know to be associated with obesity, and you know what? Nothing happened – there were no mass risings of obesity that some might describe as being 'of epidemic proportion'. That's because the environment wasn't there to switch on the genes that predispose to putting on body fat. And even this switching of genes associated with obesity we now know to be complex and seemingly contradictory – it's not just the environment that you experience, but the environments that your mother and grandmother experienced in the past that are important. Let me explain.

There often wasn't enough food to go round in the past, either all of the time or some of the time, and so our ancestors adapted by switching genes on or off, in anticipation of future need of their function. Such gene switching in relation to environment through biochemical capping or uncapping – epigenetics – created predispositions to obesity in subsequent generations. Obesity became a middle-class problem when the problems of getting enough food largely came under control in the later part of the twentieth century – when genes now known to be associated with body fatness and obesity could finally switch on (frequently aided by gene expression promoted by maternal and grand-maternal undernutrition) on a regular basis among many people. Following the rapid growth of obesity in the Global North, obesity began to grow quickly in the Global South and elsewhere, when environments predisposing to obesity started to emerge.

That's an over-simplified narrative, partly because obesity and type 2 diabetes had already been seen in some places in the Global South prior to the expansion of obesity in the Global North.

In the evolutionary past, the genetics associated with obesity now would then have been for survival, for scavenging energy from what food was available, not obesity. The people best at that, with their genetically underpinned efficient metabolism, survived, reproduced and passed on their genes for efficient metabolism to the next generation. And on to the generation after, and the one after that, and on and on, as long as these genetic adaptations continued to be useful for survival and reproduction. This was hard-won, the genetics for surviving food deprivation, as have been the epigenetic and developmental modifiers of this genetics. These genetic and developmental adaptations for survival in lean food times are the very same ones that predispose to obesity in present-day times and places of food plenty, and this is what I consider now.

How Do Genes for Survival Become Genetics of Obesity?

Obesity may never have existed in human evolutionary history except in individuals with unusual genetics, such as those found in people with monogenic forms of obesity now. As obesity is a relatively recent issue in human history, too recent for our genetics to have changed much, some scholars, most famously James Neel, of the University of Michigan, surmised in the early 1960s that genes that were adaptive in the past and that helped us be a successful species became maladaptive only in the past several decades. His thrifty gene hypothesis concerned the genetics of type 2 diabetes in modernizing populations of the Global South, but was subsequently extended to include obesity genetics. Neel's hypothesis offers an adaptive basis for having the genetic predisposition for storing masses of fat in adipose tissue (Chapter 1) when circumstances allow it, to buffer against shortfalls in dietary energy in lean times. People practising non-industrial agriculture often still go through seasonal cycles of food plenty and food shortages, and being able to store dietary energy efficiently in and on the body in times of plenty protects them against starvation in the lean times. In the absence of cycles of food availability, they would be more disposed to gaining body fat without subsequently losing it, potentially leading to obesity. In places like the Pacific, across prehistory, people had to deal with the adaptive challenge of surviving long voyages across the ocean, facing multiple stresses across generations as human populations radiated across the islands. It was the people who were best able to get the most metabolic energy from their food that were best placed to survive. Using Neel's framing, genetic adaptations for more efficient metabolism among Pacific Islanders and Native Americans were viewed by researchers as perhaps being enriched, and this is one reason why considerable research into diabetes and obesity genetics has been carried out among such groups.

The thrifty gene hypothesis views human genetics as being likely to have undergone natural selection for aspects of physiology and behaviour that promote energy intake and storage, while minimizing energy expenditure. Exactly when in prehistory such adaptation would have happened is difficult to know. What we do know is that there is great diversity in obesity-related genotypes, with the vast majority being related to more than one gene locus, usually many. All aspects of metabolism are under genetic control, and the expression of obesity phenotypes is much more limited than the expression of the enzymes and other protein factors that regulate metabolism. So it is likely that natural selection for the capacity to save and store energy would have taken place differently in different populations for different genes and gene-regions, with similar body size and overall fatness outcomes. Neel himself thought something like this – that many different genes underwent natural selection in different populations and geographic areas and under different kinds of environmental pressures, resulting in great diversity in obesity genetics.

The thrifty gene hypothesis is an imperfect descriptor of the rise in obesity in indigenous populations and has undergone modification across the past few decades to include schema such as syndromes of impaired genetic homeostasis, civilization syndromes, and altered lifestyle syndromes. Alternative views of evolution and natural selection have enriched or challenged Neel's hypothesis. In the late 2000s, John Speakman, of the University of Aberdeen, put forward his 'drifty genotype' idea of obesity, suggesting that most mutations in obesity susceptibility genes could have been neutral, having drifted over evolutionary time, rather than having been selected for. This is based on the neutral theory of evolution, by Motoo Kimura, of the National Institute of Genetics, Mishima, published in 1968. An alternative perspective, from Speakman again, is that of maladaptation – in which he suggests that genes that predispose to obesity may have been favoured as maladaptive by-products of positive natural selection for some other advantageous trait. A possible example of this might be for differences in brown adipose tissue (BAT) content and composition due to differential exposure of ancestral modern humans to cold, hot and temperature-seasonal environments. BAT is able to generate heat by burning metabolic energy to maintain body temperature under cold conditions (Chapter 3). Genetics controlling the development and expression of this tissue would have been important in the evolutionary past because they would have favoured survival by controlling thermoregulation, especially among newborn and young children. A gene essential for body temperature maintenance in cold climates is *UCP1*, encoding uncoupling protein 1, which is highly expressed in BAT (more about this later, and in Chapter 3). John Speakman subsequently elaborated his drifty gene hypothesis by adding predation release, or the removal of predation stress among early hominins, to it.

How does this idea work? According to Speakman, early hominins would have been subjected to stabilizing selection for body fatness, natural selection resulting in reduced genetic diversity as populations stabilized around particular physical and physiological traits that were of benefit to them – in this context, obesity would have been selected against by the risk of predation. But around 2 million years ago, predation was removed as a selection pressure by the development of social behaviour, weapons and fire. Greater body fatness would no longer have been selected against by predation, and there would have been a change in genetic predispositions to population distribution of body fatness through genetic drift.

Another evolutionary explanation, related to BAT activity, is the thermogenesis hypothesis of Dyan Sellayah, of the University of Reading. In this framing, migration of human populations in prehistory out of Africa and into higher latitudes would have resulted in evolution of more efficient BAT activity and *UCP1*, leading to populations in cold climates burning more energy for maintaining body temperature than populations in warm climates, giving them a higher metabolic rate which could have lowered predispositions to obesity.

A key environmental stressor in the evolutionary past would have been food seasonality (Chapter 7), overeating when food was plentiful, depositing body fat to tide over the hungry times. Humans and other mammals will overeat and put on body fat when presented with diets that are plentiful, palatable, and/or high in fat, suggesting that the tendency to overeat in response to food-portion size, palatability, and energy density, and to overeat fat passively are general mammalian evolutionary traits. Most mammals are able to overeat to high levels of body fatness, suggesting that some of the genetic basis for human obesity must lie in evolutionary time that is deeper than that of the hominin–chimpanzee divergence of over 7 million years ago. In addition, social aspects of feeding are also common across species; for example, social interaction during eating increases food intake in chickens and apes, as well as among humans.

Right now, the jury is out as to which of these ideas concerning the evolution of traits that can lead to obesity is right – are they the genetics for survival? Is it sheer bad luck they survive in us now, when we need to resist calorie intake and efficient metabolism if we want to avoid gaining significant body weight? There is no way of knowing what really happened in hominin evolution, although some inferences can be made. Thrift and drift are known to operate in evolution more broadly, and it is likely that both thrifty and drifty genetics are implicated in the production of human obesity. Predation release and thermogenesis are also very plausible ideas, but what is missing is an integrated view of how genetics related to obesity might have co-evolved.

A Short History of Genetics and Obesity

The idea that obesity may have a genetic basis is almost as old as Mendelian genetics itself. In 1907, medical doctor Carl von Noorden, then at the University of Vienna, classified obesity into two types, exogenous and endogenous. The exogenous form of obesity was considered by him to be the consequence of external factors such as excessive food consumption (the physiology of overeating was little known then, and was not considered to be due to internal, or endogenous factors). Endogenous obesity was seen as being usually caused by physiological disorders such as hypometabolism or other thyroid disorders, and was taken to be innate or, in present-day terms, genetic. The word 'gene' was coined in 1909 by Wilhelm Johanssen, a botanist at the Royal Veterinary and Agricultural College in Copenhagen, who went on to define the terms 'genotype' and 'phenotype', as a way of distinguishing the hereditary dispositions of organisms and the ways in which they manifest themselves in the physical characteristics of those organisms. In relation to obesity, the genotype was simply the hereditary disposition to put on excess weight, and it wasn't thought about much, if at all, for nearly 50 years, until James Neel's time.

Although the double helix structure of DNA was identified in the 1950s, the new genetics that emerged from this work didn't see obesity as an object for research, probably because obesity wasn't a pressing medical problem at that time. The shift to modern genetics thinking in obesity science was initiated by Neel in the 1960s. Obesity genes, as meaningful stretches of DNA that code for enzymes and other proteins that mediate fat deposition, had not been identified, but Neel thought that there must be genes to be discovered that predispose to type 2 diabetes and to obesity. Such genes were thought by Neel to have been advantageous to individuals and populations in the past, but becoming detrimental as the world modernized and food security became increasingly assured for much of the world's population. By the end of the 1970s, high rates of type 2 diabetes in combination with obesity had been observed in populations outside the Euro-American mainstream, on Samoa and the Cook Islands, and in remote-dwelling Indigenous Australians. These were all populations that had undergone dietary change, with increased consumption of refined carbohydrates, sugar especially. How this diet change came about, often through colonial coercion and destruction of the traditional food ways of such groups, is a less often told narrative among medics and geneticists researching obesity.

In the 1980s, a number of adoption and twin studies were carried out by Albert Stunkard and colleagues at the University of Pennsylvania, Philadelphia, and elsewhere. Stunkard and colleagues found that the body weights of adult twins reared in an adopted family were closer to their biological parents than to their adoptive parents, indicating a strong genetic component to body size (including fatness) and obesity. They also found that the heritability of BMI, from measures of twins reared together and apart, was between 40 and 70 per cent. That is, of the differences in BMI within any population, a very considerable proportion of such difference was inherited. Around the same time, DNA-based genetics research into obesity took off, initially involving understanding of the genetics of energy balance through monogenic mouse and rat models of obesity, with a focus on the genes for leptin (*LEP*), the leptin receptor (*LEPR*), and the agouti gene and agouti-related protein. The hormone leptin acts on the brain to regulate appetite and several other physiological functions, while the leptin receptor is found in tissues across the body but especially the brain, allowing the expression of chemical signals that do several jobs at the cellular level – regulating appetite in the brain, but also regulating reproduction and a broad range of metabolic processes. The agouti gene and agouti-related protein regulate energy metabolism and the control of body weight. What followed in the 1990s was the identification of people with congenital leptin deficiency, and subsequently people with mutations in *LEPR*, and in genes encoding the appetite-regulating melanocortin pathway.

Layering complexity onto the thrifty gene hypothesis, type 2 diabetes, obesity, and hypertension were bundled together into so-called 'syndromes of impaired genetic homeostasis', 'civilization syndromes', and 'altered lifestyle syndromes'. The modified thrifty gene hypothesis came to include the tendency to overeat as well as obesity; and the environments in which the tendency to overeat presented itself were subsequently described as being obesogenic (about which more is said in Chapter 7).

As gene-tech progressed in the 2000s, high-throughput DNA sequencing (in which many segments of DNA are sequenced in parallel, generating much more data much more quickly) led to candidate gene screening being replaced by approaches that allowed all coding sequences of DNA to be screened for mutations. The first human genome was sequenced in 1990, and the hunt intensified for the genetics of obesity and of many diseases associated with it. As evidence of genes associated with body size (usually the BMI), appetite and energy expenditures amassed, so a directory of obesity-related genes was initiated in 1994. Soon after, this regularly updated directory became known as the obesity gene map directory. By 2005, human obesity due to single-gene mutations in 11 different genes had been identified. Fifty loci related to Mendelian syndromes relevant to human obesity had been mapped to a genomic region, with causal genes or strong genetic candidates having been identified for most of these syndromes. Research that followed included the mapping of quantitative trait loci (QTLs) for body size. Obesity-related QTLs are genetic regions that influence variation in some aspect associated with obesity. In general, QTLs are seen to do their work directly but also through genetic interactions with each other and with the environment. By the late 2000s, the number of QTLs reported from animal models exceeded 400, with over 250 human obesity-related QTLs having been identified from over 60 genome scans. No longer looking directly for genes associated with body fatness or obesity, genome scanning allowed the systematic scanning of the entire DNA for locations on the genetic material that are inherited similarly to the obesity-related traits under investigation. Of the 250-plus human obesity-related QTLs, over 50 genomic regions were confirmed by two or more studies, making them clear candidates for further investigation. The number of studies reporting associations between DNA sequence variation in specific genes and obesity phenotypes increased, with over 400 findings of positive associations with over 120 candidate genes. The obesity gene map showed putative loci on all chromosomes except Y, itself containing the *SRY* gene that determines whether an embryo will develop as a male (XY) or a female (XX), but very little else of importance.

As the number of genes and genomic regions associated with obesity rose, researchers increasingly homed in on most likely candidates for common obesity. The rare, monogenic types had been largely characterized by 2005, but they could only explain 4 per cent of all population-level obesity. The search for common genetic variants led to the identification of three genes as being especially important for the development of common obesity. The fat mass and obesity-associated (*FTO*) gene was identified by Tim Frayling of the University of Exeter and his many collaborators in 2007, from a genome-wide association (GWA) study for type 2 diabetes, revealing *FTO* to be an obesity-related gene instead. Another GWA study of 17,000 subjects, published in 2009, identified common variants in the *MC4R* gene associated with BMI, while a third study identified the *PCSK1* gene as a strong common obesity gene candidate. All three were viewed as being involved in hypothalamic regulation, but each only explained a very tiny proportion of all obesity. A hopeful reason given by scientists for this low explanatory value was their expectation that a huge number of additional genes and gene areas must all contribute to obesity but had not been picked up in studies that were searching for common genes. As more genes and genetic regions were identified as being linked to obesity, some research turned back to consider how much, collectively, the many genes of very small effect might contribute to the overall heritability of obesity. One such analysis was that of Jian Yang, of the Queensland Institute of Medical Research, and his many colleagues, which was published in 2011. The additive effects of over half a million single-nucleotide polymorphisms (single DNA base-pair variants) were genotyped for over 10,000 unrelated individuals, but despite the large scale of this hugely ambitious project, the results were sobering. These researchers succeeded in collectively explaining only 17 per cent of the population variance in BMI, falling far short of the known range of heritability from adoption and twin studies (of between 40 and 70 per cent for BMI). A genetic model of obesity should be able to account for these levels of variance, if the effect is really directly genetic.

So Where Are We Now?

The past decade has seen an explosion of GWA studies of common obesity phenotypes, but all that has been revealed is that their effects on fat mass are so small that it is hard to definitively establish the impact of each individual variant on food intake, energy expenditure, or energy partitioning. This is with one exception, the *FTO* gene, where carriers of the risk allele have consistently been reported to have a strong relationship with appetite and/or high objectively measured food intakes. In a critical review of the obesity genetics literature, Ruth Loos and Giles Yeo, of the Mount Sinai School of Medicine, New York, and the University of Cambridge, respectively, see obesity genetics as still falling into one of two categories, monogenic and polygenic, even after decades of obesity genetics research that has allowed these categories to be questioned thoroughly. This typology is a refinement, over a hundred years later, of Carl von Noorden's initial classification of obesity into two types, endogenous and exogenous, or innate and externally stimulated obesity. Jean-Baptiste Alphonse Karr wrote to the effect that the more that things change, the more they stay the same. Genetics didn't exist as a subject when he wrote that in 1849, but it seems to apply to obesity genetics – over a hundred years since the terms 'genotype' and 'phenotype' were coined by Wilhelm Johanssen, they continue to be used in much the same way as they were initially defined. Monogenic obesity is inherited in a Mendelian pattern, is typically rare, early-onset, severe, and involves chromosomal deletions or single-gene defects. Polygenic obesity (also known as common obesity) is the result of hundreds of polymorphisms that each have a small effect, but that require obesogenic environmental stimulus. While there has been no revolution in thinking about obesity typologies, physiological research into both types of obesity has shown them to have broadly similar underlying biology. This is considered further in Chapter 3.

The missing heritability in obesity genetics has led to calls for ever-larger and more intricate study designs to 'find the gap'. A huge gap in fact, of between a fifth and a half of overall variance in measures of obesity and its proxies. It is possible that this gap may be due not to not-yet-identified genes and genomic regions with very small influence on obesity, but to the expression of already known genes and gene regions and their interactions. Predispositions to obesity are not just genetic, but also epigenetic and developmental. The term 'epigenetics' was coined in 1942 by Conrad Waddington, an embryologist then at the University of Cambridge, who, relating it to the seventeenth-century concept of epigenesis, defined it as the complex of developmental processes between the genotype and phenotype. In the age of DNA, it has come to mean changes in gene activity not involving changes in DNA sequence – how changes to the structure of DNA molecules can alter the expression of genes. Priyadarshni Patel and her colleagues at Auburn University, Alabama, together with the Hudson Alpha Institute for Biotechnology, have reviewed research into epigenetic expression of obesity-related genes, mostly in animal models but also in humans, and especially in relation to macronutrient intake. They conclude that while such work is persuasive of a link between diet and expression of genetics associated with obesity in animal models, research in humans is more limited and suggestive.

In obesity research, the idea of epigenetics was primed by the 'fetal origins' hypothesis of David Barker, then of the Medical Research Council Environmental Epidemiology Unit, Southampton, which established the notion of metabolic programming, in which nutritional and other exposures during early life are seen to generate long-term changes that later predispose to type 2 diabetes and cardiovascular disease. This hypothesis built on epidemiology research that showed strong links between early life events, most commonly in-utero, and disease risk in later adult life. A vivid example of this comes from research on health in later life among those born in, or soon after, the Dutch Famine of 1944–45. At its peak in the first months of 1945, the official daily ration for the general population varied between 400 and 800 calories, virtually a starvation diet. Hospitals and clinics carried on their services, reporting and recording maternal and young child health, then in the context of severe food insecurity. Following up 50 years later, Anita Ravelli, and colleagues at the Universities of Southampton and Amsterdam, found that daughters of women who had gone through early pregnancy during this period of starvation were more likely to be considered overweight than those who had been born to women after the famine. Epigenetic processes are strong candidates for mediating this effect, and data from the Dutch Famine offered a big opportunity to determine this, once epigenetic research protocols for studying DNA methylation and demethylation had been put in place. Research confirmed epigenetic changes affecting growth, metabolic disease, and obesity predisposition in these daughters. It also confirmed the intrauterine environment to be an important predisposer to obesity, agreeing in largest part with observational studies that offspring obesity and fatness relationships are greater for mothers than for fathers.

Following this, Oyvind Helgeland, of the Norwegian Institute of Public Health, and his colleagues in Bergen, Oslo, Trondheim and Gothenberg recently carried out a study of the genetic architecture of BMI in infancy and early childhood, showing age-specific effects. They grouped genetic associations with early BMI into three main clusters that align with phases of early child growth. These are: a birth cluster, characterized by loci mainly acting on fetal growth; a transient and an early-rise cluster, which influences BMI during transitions around a peak of adiposity and its rebound; and a late-rise cluster of loci, which come into play later in childhood and have persistent influence on BMI into adult life. They suggest that BMI in childhood is shaped by a complex interplay of transitions from both age-restricted and longer-term genetic influences which should be taken into consideration when evaluating a child's growth pattern and the potential for targeted interventions against obesity. Thus, while early development of excess body fatness might appear to be of clinical importance, it may be so for reasons other than the long-term development of obesity. More important for the development of obesity into adult life is child growth from the period of adiposity rebound (a rise in body mass index that occurs between 3 and 7 years) and just before onset of puberty.

After the identification of *FTO* as the only gene of major effect associated with common obesity, it was found that this effect is attenuated by physical activity, diet, and drug-based interventions. In the original *FTO* study, 16 per cent of nearly 39,000 study participants carried this obesity-related gene variant, making the overall population variance in obesity rate due to *FTO* around 10 per cent of all obesity. If obesity rates in the population are 30 per cent, then *FTO* might explain 3 per cent of overall obesity rate in that population – still very small, but as big as it gets for common obesity. Epigenetic modification has since been shown to influence the expression of the *FTO* gene, and thus its link to obesity. Both diet and physical activity modulate DNA methylation more broadly, offering a mechanistic link to both of these factors and the development of chronic disease. Thus, epigenetic modification may be a key link between environment and genetics in the production (or not) of obesity.

What Can We Do?

Understanding the evolutionary processes that lead to obesity predisposition in the general population is useful for medical and public health intervention, in two ways. First, separating monogenic from common obesity allows clinical and treatment regimes to be followed for the former, focusing on the identification of the gene involved, followed by gene-specific treatment. Such treatment functions by increasing or decreasing levels of circulating gene products to promote lipolysis and increasing energy expenditure, with an ultimate aim of reducing body fatness. It is administered by targeted delivery of therapeutic genes to specific cells, causing increased expression of gene products that promote weight loss. A number of genes associated with monogenic obesity are targets for treatment. These include leptin-replacement treatment for *LEP* deficiency and *MC4R* agonists for *LEPR*, *PCSK1*, and *POMC* deficiency. Second, with respect to common obesity, an integrated view of how some common genes that are related to obesity might have evolved would be useful for framing public health responses to it. Whether thrifty, drifty, predation release, or BAT-related, each offers different but overlapping understandings of common obesity in the present day. Thrifty and drifty gene framings offer different ways of thinking about evolutionary processes in developing predispositions to common obesity. Predation release would have accelerated genetic driftiness. Prehistoric human migrations from tropical climes and into colder ones would have allowed the evolution of more efficient BAT activity, higher metabolic rate, increased energy expenditure, and lower predispositions to obesity.

Obesity genotypes and energy balance susceptibilities to obesity can only be expressed in positive energy ecologies, where it is easy for energy intake to exceed energy expenditure, and/or when energy intake is dominated by refined carbohydrate. Such ecologies have been vaguely defined as obesogenic environments, or environments that predispose to obesity. According to Harry Rutter, of the University of Bath, increasing fatness is a result of a normal response, by normal people, to an abnormal situation. The abnormal situation is the present-day world and how people negotiate it, about which more will be said in Chapters 4 and 5. The abnormal situation is largely structural, put in place at an earlier time when food security could not be guaranteed, before the global rise in obesity. You can't change your genetics, but you might think about how the abnormal world we live in could be adjusted so that genetic predispositions to common obesity are not realized. Now, if you can't fit into your skinny jeans any more, you can't just blame your genes – at least most people can't. Like me, you might just be older, not wiser, but wider than you were in your twenties.

From a policy perspective, maternal and grand-maternal histories may well shape present-day likelihoods of developing obesity. Appropriate nutrition in pregnancy and during child development are key to health at all stages of life, and policy focused on maternal health and child-centred social investment would help to reduce the legacy of obesity and chronic disease created by past political, economic, and social environments in countries of the Global North embracing market liberalism.

At the level of the individual, how can knowledge of genetics of obesity help you, and, if you have genetics that predispose to obesity, your children? Knowing that the genetic underpinning of common obesity affects most people should help to take the spotlight off personal responsibility, in as far as people with obesity are discriminated against and stigmatized (Chapter 6). With respect to individual treatment, there are many candidates for gene therapy against obesity, but these are overwhelmingly focused on fixing monogenic obesity. An exception to this is work on clock machinery genes associated with circadian rhythm. Sleeping well and having adequate exposure to daylight both influence body weight regulation, and this ought to help. Research into *FTO* gene therapeutics is now a candidate, since a link has been found between *FTO* and breast cancer, offering a new target for cancer gene therapy. The primary role of *FTO* is in the sensing of macronutrients, and it would not be surprising if it is also linked to type 2 diabetes. The major methods of gene therapy are viral, with non-viral delivery carrier systems targeting appropriate tissues. For the time being, these remain part of the promissory landscape of gene therapy more broadly. Epigenetics might offer an alternative to gene therapy. Altered methylation can modify gene expression, which can in turn translate into changes in cellular pathways and phenotypes. Many studies have reported associations between DNA methylation levels and hundreds of human diseases and traits. Cancer is also at the forefront of epigenetic-targeted therapy research, and this might offer another approach for developing obesity treatment. Finally, genetics and epigenetics offer evidence that your ancestry matters, with your deeply inherited biological background, as does the life experience of your mother and possibly your grandmother, in your likelihood of gaining excess weight in adult life.

3 It's My Metabolism

Driving on Life's Freeway

Some people talk of their metabolism like they might talk of the performance of a motor car – slow or fast. Many people carrying excess weight might like to attribute it to their slow metabolism, but there's no evidence that it works that way. In fact, there is evidence that metabolism is neither slow nor fast, but varies across a gradient both within and between populations. A small number of people are at the upper end of this gradient and are much less likely to gain excess weight than the small number of people who are at the lower end. There are also some people who do have genuinely very slow metabolism, but this is usually down to them having an endocrine or metabolic disorder. But driving on life's metabolic freeway, most people are neither crawling in the slow lane nor cruising in the fast lane, but changing lanes according to circumstance. Like freeway driving, metabolism is dynamic, flexible, and adaptable.

In this chapter I talk about energy metabolism as it relates to obesity, describing various models of this mechanism, as well as the ways in which thinking in this field has changed since the 1950s. I discuss how natural selection for the ability to save and store energy as body fat probably took place for a range of genetics, ultimately to the same effect. Obesity, metabolism, and the brain are intricately interconnected, and so I go on to consider the neurobiology of obesity from an evolutionary perspective: that is, why this physiological system should have made us so successful in surviving the hardships of life prior to the age we live in, and why this system is now a curse in the present age of food plenty. I finish by discussing how the tight feedback loops of metabolism make it difficult to intervene in the regulation of body weight in any simple way, at least for now.

Without Metabolism, We Would Be Dead – So What Is Metabolism?

According to my University of Oxford colleague Professor Keith Frayn, who recently wrote an excellent companion book in this series, called *Understanding Metabolism*, it's not so simple – everyone has a metabolism, but then so does everything alive on this planet. Its early evolution set the conditions for all aspects of life, from single-celled organisms to highly coordinated complex multicellular ones like ourselves. Nearly everything in our bodies is made through metabolic processes, and the processes that keep us alive are metabolism too. No exaggeration, without metabolism, we would be dead. The most active metabolic processes are those that convert nutrients from foods we eat into the building materials of our cells and tissues as well as generating ATP – adenosine triphosphate. And to a lesser extent GTP – guanosine triphosphate. I think of ATP as the gasoline that fuels all the processes that keep us alive. But unlike in an old-style motor car, we can't store much ATP in our bodies. We don't have an ATP tank that we can fill up when it runs low. No, we make it as we go along, from energy-containing foods, and from bodily tissues when we haven't eaten or been able to eat. The closest we have to a gas-tank is our adipose tissue, which isn't really a tank at all. I talk about adipose tissue in Chapter 1 – most of it either surrounds the gut or is overcoat-like external fat around the outside of the body, especially around the trunk, buttocks, and thighs. If a car were more like us, what would it look like? One of artist Erwin Wurm's fat cars may give you an idea (Figure 3.1).

Unlike Wurm's Fat Car, our bodies are constantly monitoring, depositing, and withdrawing fat from both internal and external adipose tissue. We need some level of body fat to live, survive, and thrive, of that there is no doubt. But it only becomes a problem for health when we accumulate enough in the adipose tissue that it pushes our metabolism towards illnesses like type 2 diabetes, cardiovascular disease, and some cancers. Altered metabolism is also one of the reasons why people with severe obesity came down more heavily with COVID-19 infection in the early months of the 2020 pandemic. The old-style motor car has a fuel tank of a certain size, non-negotiably so. Our bodies differ

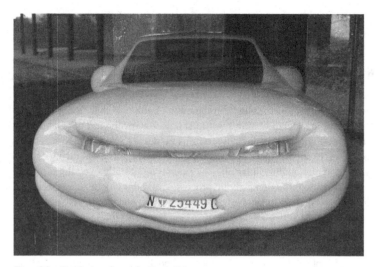

Figure 3.1 'Fat Car' sculpture by Erwin Wurm.

again, in that adipose tissue can grow and expand to the point of our physical immobility, if we let it. The constant monitoring, depositing, and withdrawing of fat is what most people talk about when they talk about metabolism and obesity. This is the idea of energy balance, about how the body regulates what comes in through food – energy intake – and what goes out through bodily development, maintenance, and physical activity – energy expenditure.

What goes out, energy expenditure, comprises energy spent in bodily maintenance, physical activity, digesting food, and in keeping us warm. It's a bit like a bank account, with food energy coming in being the paycheck, and energy expenditure being your payments, except that the direct debits are not exactly the same every month, nor is income. One thing that is in constant flux is how much ATP we make and how much we use in energy expenditure. As with income and expenditure, some people have a steadier relationship with energy than others. And at a social and political level, energy balance, and obesity, relate to financial well-being (or not) – more about this in Chapter 5. Some aspects of energy expenditure can vary a lot according to changing circumstances, and the energy exchange rate also varies according to whether you are eating heartily or poorly, whether you are physically active or not, and even what kinds of foods you get your dietary energy from. And the aim at the end of any period is not to have a positive bank balance – these days, putting energy in the Bank of the Body usually does you no good beyond a certain level.

The Bank of the Body trades mostly in the currency of adipose tissue, and can deposit it in several places, which, unlike shifting your money into a deposit account, you have little control over. If my bank did this to me, I would switch to one that gave me more control. Unfortunately, the Bank of the Body is yours for life, no switching, no changing. But the body, and metabolism, do not respond similarly to different sources of dietary energy. More about this, and the alternative carbohydrate–insulin model of obesity, later in this Chapter, and in Chapter 7.

You might have heard of homeostasis, how the body's physiology stays in balance. In the case of body fatness, this involves many metabolic checks and balances involved in matching energy intake through the food we eat to the energy we expend (Figure 3.2). When intake exceeds expenditure, positive

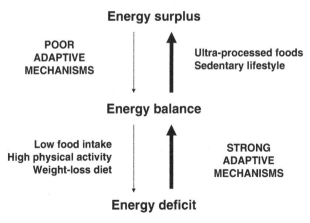

Figure 3.2 Physiological homeostasis and weight regulation.

energy balance can lead to deposition of fat, and the body can be seen as being out of homeostasis when this happens; when we lose body fat if we eat less than we burn, then this is being out of homeostasis too. The idea of homeostasis comes from thinking in ancient Greece, with the doctrine of balance of opposite qualities. In obesity science, ideas of physiological homeostasis and energy balance are used interchangeably, as both are concerned with energy flow through living systems by the process of metabolism, or energy transformation within biological systems.

We eat, we sleep, we work, we love, we mate, we live, and all the time our metabolism allows us to do all of these things, almost without us having to think about them. We make decisions, though, about what to eat, how to eat, with whom to eat, how we get to work (or not), and what we do in leisure time. Well, many of us do – income and where you live matters, and there is no denying that in wealthy countries the cheapest, energy-dense food is often the worst for us, and is most concentrated in poorer neighbourhoods. More about these issues in Chapters 4 and 5. Eating, drinking, walking, running, sleeping, thinking, all these things get integrated in a metabolic bottom line, with homeostasis being maintained (or not) over shorter and longer time intervals. We can't really see short-term physiological homeostasis – most usually, metabolic scientists are the only ones that have privileged access to this, in their laboratories. Free-living humans, like all other mammals, show only a semblance of longer-term energy homeostasis. And this is only if the non-homeostatic processes of reproduction and physical growth and development are ignored. Ultimately, metabolism underpins the evolutionary success of a species through reproductive success, but this is usually ignored for the purposes of trying to understand energy balance in relation to obesity.

Decades of study have shown the relationships between energy intake and expenditure to be both complex and intertwined, and many of us personally experience the cruel hand of metabolic fate when trying to lose weight. It can be so very difficult to lose the weight we put on over Christmas and other times of repeated feasting, in time for summer holidays when we might aspire to show off trim healthy bodies. The cruel truth of homeostasis is that it exists to serve evolutionary processes, and its physiological mechanisms defend the body against changes in energy balance. In this sense, it is so much more sophisticated than the fuel injection system of the most elegant Ferrari motor car.

Across months and years, energy brought into the body by eating food must balance energy expended in bodily maintenance, reproduction, and physical activity (and in children, physical growth and development), to avoid either undernutrition or obesity. Human physiology is much better able to strike such a balance when there is less food available than when food is plentiful. Where getting enough food is a challenge, as in some traditional societies now and among poorer sectors of western society in the past, physiological energy deficits can lead to weight loss initially, but energy balance usually recalibrates at lower levels of intake and expenditure. This is because physiological and behavioural adaptations defend body size and composition, achieving homeostasis at lower levels of energy turnover. When food is plentiful, there are only very weak homeostatic mechanisms that can restore individual energy balance. So it is easier for your body to defend its existing size against food shortages than for it to defend against food surpluses. Eat too little, and it is not so easy to lose weight, eat too much and it is easy to put it on. This may sound familiar to you, if you have tried a weight-loss diet involving food restriction – weight loss is hard-earned, while weight gain can happen so easily and without thinking. I will talk more about this in Chapter 7, when I discuss food intake and cognitive restraint.

Metabolism and Genetics

Since metabolism involves biochemical processes that require enzymes to catalyse them, much of what underpins metabolism therefore has a genetic basis – that is, genes, or gene-regions that code for proteins, many of which are enzymes involved in metabolism. The mundane, everyday chemical reactions of metabolism take place in all of the cells of the body, which, in relation to energetics, convert food energy into chemical energy, ultimately ATP, which is used for running all the bodily processes. Unlike the old-style motor car, these chemical processes happen at body temperature, driven by enzymes, which, as we've said, are proteins coded by genes. There is little surprise then that some genetic mutations that cause errors in metabolism are associated with metabolic disorders, some of them associated with obesity. Metabolic disorders fall into two broad categories, those that are inherited, and those that are acquired. The former come from inborn errors of metabolism, due to genetic defects in coding for proteins, usually enzymes associated with metabolism, and these can lead to several possible metabolic disorders, including ones associated with lysosomal storage in white adipose tissue (WAT) and the liver. Lysosomes are organelles within cells that can break down long molecules like proteins, carbohydrates, and fats, for recycling in the body. Metabolic disorders associated with lysosomal storage are linked to a cluster of conditions that associate with obesity and occur together, increasing the likelihood of developing heart disease, stroke, and type 2 diabetes. Metabolic syndrome is an acquired metabolic disorder associated with external factors, including poor diet, high energy intake, and leading a sedentary life. Epigenetics can play its part in this, with altered gene expression (see Chapter 2), which can alter the activity of enzymes and other proteins involved in metabolism, which in turn can lead to the development of metabolic diseases or disorders.

The genetics of metabolism is important, but complicated. The field of metabolomics has helped unravel some of the issues involved. Gabi Kastenmuller and her colleagues, at the Institute of Bioinformatics and Systems Biology at the Helmholtz Zentrum in Munich, have applied genome-wide association studies with metabolomics (mGWAS) to show just how interconnected the genetic regulation of energy metabolism really is. These interconnections are powerful, enmeshed, keeping time's arrow of metabolism moving on life's freeway.

The Physiology of How Obesity Is Developed – Some Models

Since the emergence of obesity as a population-level issue, many scientists have developed models to help explain its causation, emergence, and rapid increase. These include models that invoke thrifty genotypes, genomics, eating behaviour, obesogenic environments, ecology, nutrition transition, and epigenetics, as well as integrated models that examine interactions of some or many of these factors. All obesity models are just that, models. British statistician George E. P. Box famously wrote, in 1976, that "All models are wrong, but some are useful." Which is to say that they are imperfect representations of reality. They fall into two broad types – 'models of', and 'models for'. A model of something, like a map, attempts to represent that something. Like with any topographical map, decisions need to be made by the modeller on what is important to keep in and leave out. According to its use, some things are more important than others – Google Maps, for example, usually leaves out altitude and hill contours, but includes quite detailed road systems. Alternatively, a 'model for' is for problem-solving (analytical problem-solving models are widespread in business and science). A model for obesity intervention and its regulation should include things that can be acted upon. Different things are incorporated into a model for obesity, according to whether it is being used for treatment, for epidemiological monitoring, for public health intervention, for economic policy. No 'model for' can hope to represent that totality of a phenomenon, but it should help us think or through an issue towards an action. All models (of, for) inevitably reveal very partial truths, and are conditional on the science of the moment. New research can either validate or change a model, but models are important for putting into order what is known about obesity at a given time, and working out what still needs to be known, what can be acted upon, and how. Models of, and for, obesity come together in building the science to a point where new forms of intervention, policy or prevention can be put forward with confidence.

Models of obesity do mostly representational work, for the understanding and prediction of cause-and-effect relationships, for example, in energy balance or in carbohydrate intake and insulin response. Although obesity has been problematized in many ways, the dominant frameworks are medical, public health, and economic, all of them mostly based on the energy-balance model of obesity. There are, however, several models which relate the structuring of energy intake and expenditure to individual physiological regulation of energy input and output at the whole-body level, that incorporate or are based in metabolism. Here are some of the more important ones.

The set-point model was well developed by the 1980s and is based on epidemiological observations that show that many people have more or less constant body weight across adult life. It views body weight and body fatness as being kept in homeostasis by internal hormonal regulation. Tests of this model show the set point in humans to have upper and lower limits, rather than being under tight control. Fluctuations in body weight that come from experimental under- or overfeeding need to be big to shift the theoretical set point in any individual. The model seems to work quite well under experimental conditions when subjects eat boring but healthy chow diets, but real life is not a metabolic feeding laboratory. Take the model out into the world you and I live in, with its supermarket discounts, sandwich shops with their meal-deals, and cheap-as-chips fried chicken shops, and it starts to unravel. The strong biological control of body weight and weight stability that the set-point model predicts is easily overwhelmed when people eat the more palatable energy-dense diets available to them now. Another issue with this model is that demonstrating clear set points in different people is difficult to do, so it has been modified to try to account for this. There are now several modifications of the set-point idea, making it less and less useful as a model for obesity intervention. It might not actually be how energy metabolism works.

Stephen Simpson and David Raubenheimer, both at the University of Sydney, think not. They have proposed an alternative to the set-point model, the protein leverage hypothesis. The logic for this is as follows. The macronutrient composition of diet and its effects on satiation (physiological cues to terminate eating) and satiety (the feeling of fullness after eating) can vary enormously both within a person and between people. High-fat foods have weak effects on satiation and satiety compared with refined carbohydrates, while protein has the strongest effect on both. Energy-dense, fat-rich foods (such as the ultra-processed foods described in Chapter 4) have been shown to give less satiation and satiety than more bulky, hydrated foods that are high in protein, fibre, or water content. That is, mostly fruit and vegetables, as well as protein-rich foods, to you and me. In general, diets that are more energy-dense have lower effects on satiation and satiety, making it easier to overeat passively and gain weight. Low protein content in an otherwise energy-rich diet also encourages overeating. When humans trade off their protein intake against carbohydrate and fat on nutritionally unbalanced diets, physiological regulation of food intake prioritizes protein, so you stay hungry and keep eating until your protein needs are met. Think about this if you are ever inclined to eat a bag of potato chips, crisps, or similar salty fatty snacks. Can you satisfy your hunger with a grab-size bag of chips? The answer is an obvious 'no'. It might have nearly 250 calories, but less than 5 per cent of them come from protein. According to the protein leverage hypothesis, you might need to eat 10 of them to stop feeling hungry at one sitting, by which time you will have eaten most of your daily calorie intake at one go. And you probably won't feel good for having done it. Extending this idea to the world, Simpson and Raubenheimer argue that changing patterns of fat and carbohydrate consumption in the world are driving population obesity precisely because humans seek to obtain a constant level of intake of protein, even when its density in the diet is low. Does this model seem plausible? Yes, but in a real world with all its complexity, it doesn't tell the whole story.

Another energy-balance model of obesity, ages-old but now undergoing revival, is to do with brown adipose tissue (BAT; Chapter 1). Masayuki Saito and colleagues at Hokkaido University, Sapporo, have argued that the metabolic activity of BAT in people with high levels of it increases their energy expenditure and protects them against obesity. Sapporo is a very cold place in winter – I was there in January 2023, and on a day when the highest temperature reached minus 7 degrees Celsius, it didn't surprise me that Saito and his colleagues got the idea of researching BAT there. Their research, and of several other research groups, showed how cold exposure in humans can activate metabolism in BAT, making it increase energy expenditure. And that cold exposure can induce BAT activity in adults as well as children. And that some white adipose tissue (WAT) can be stimulated to have similar activity but at a lower level, becoming so-called beige cells (such modification of WAT has been described as beige-ing). While I had already fallen in love with BAT when I worked on it in the 1980s, under Professor David Hull, one of the two researchers who discovered the function of BAT (even earlier, in the 1960s), research undertaken in the deep freeze of a Hokkaido winter has helped me love beige (adipose tissue) too. I am sure you are dying to know how BAT does its work, so here is a (relatively) short and simple account.

Babies have much more BAT than adults, and we evolved this tissue, with its ability to generate heat when exposed to cold, for survival – newborn babies are resilient to cold exposure, and the ability to switch on BAT heat production when exposed to the cold must have allowed them to live when otherwise they might have died. Dyan Sellayah has some good ideas about how this might have evolved. This heat production, technically known as non-shivering thermogenesis (NST), helps animals to recover from lethargy and, in some species, from hibernation, as well as to maintain body temperature in warm-blooded animals such as ourselves. BAT is found only in mammals, so it must have evolved alongside the evolution of mammals more generally, since around 180 million years ago. The way that BAT generates heat is through UCP1, which sits in the inner mitochondrial membrane within the cells of this type of adipose tissue. When activated, UCP1 increases the leakiness of the mitochondrial membranes of these cells, making them convert less dietary energy into ATP and to a lesser extent, GTP. This process of ATP and GTP production in the mitochondria is called oxidative phosphorylation, or OXPHOS. I was taught in school biology that for each molecule of NADH (a bigger energy-carrying molecule, intermediary between macronutrient breakdown and ATP and GTP production) that goes into OXPHOS, three molecules of ATP, for metabolic use, are made. Well, I found out much later, when working for David Hull, that it wasn't so simple. *UCP1*, when it is switched on, uncouples OXPHOS, so that less NADH is turned into ATP and GTP. What NADH chemical energy does not get turned into ATP and GTP in OXPHOS mostly gets dissipated as heat, this heat being what allows us to be warm-blooded. In BAT with *UCP1* switched on, much less NADH is converted into ATP and GTP, and much more food energy is lost as heat, so you feel warmer because fewer of the calories you have eaten have been turned into chemical energy for energy metabolism, and more have been dissipated as heat. Think about the Ferrari and Wurm's Fat Car – when you turn off the engine after a drive, it is hot because of inefficiencies of turning gasoline into motion. Metabolic inefficiency, induced by cold exposure, makes BAT generate heat. BAT generates heat in a different way too. You know that warm fuzzy feeling you get when you have eaten a big meal, usually not of salad? Well, this diet-induced thermogenesis, switched on by eating, is generated by your BAT, which is switched on by food as well.

The gene for UCP1 far pre-dates mammalian evolution, being found in fish, which neither have BAT nor are warm-blooded. Sellayah thinks it might have provided localized heat production in the tissues that really matter, like the brain (some fish have specialized heater cells in their brains, driven by *UCP1* genes switched on by cold exposure). The *UCP1* gene helped survival of fish, and across evolutionary time was probably co-opted to a more central role in maintaining body temperature as warm-blooded species emerged. *UCP1*-dependent NST would have helped evolving mammals to increase their metabolic rates by burning more energy through inefficient conversion of NADH to ATP, allowing stable body temperature independently of the external environment, and as a consequence, adaptation to a wider range of environments across the planet. Although mammals diversified and adapted to a range of ecological niches ranging from tropical to polar by around 2 million years ago, early humans would have been highly adapted to sub-Saharan African conditions, where adaptation to heat may well have been more important than cold tolerance. Several gene variants associated with NST in BAT have been identified in humans but not in other primates, suggesting that the common ancestor of non-human primates and hominins did not have a need for energy wastage gene variants that increase metabolic heat production. But, according to Sellayah, having the ability for *UCP1*-dependent NST would have been adaptive for colder environments, as early humans migrated out of Africa across the world and into more northerly latitudes.

Energy-balance models have increasingly placed the brain as the primary organ responsible for obesity. The brain integrates external signals from the food environment (more about this in Chapter 4) – hormonal, metabolic, and nervous system signals responding to the body's dynamic energy needs as well as to environmental influences, along with internal signals from peripheral organs, to control food intake. Nervous system regulation of energy balance involves afferent neurons (which bring sensory information from the world to the brain) signalling to the brain from the periphery about the state of energy stores, and efferent neurons, which carry signals from the brain to initiate an action to other parts of the body to influence energy intake through appetite, and energy expenditure through physiological mechanisms influencing basal metabolic rate, exercise and non-exercise thermogenesis, and diet-induced thermogenesis (see Chapter 1). In these ways, everyday energy intake and energy balance can vary a lot (think of a day of fasting versus a day of feasting), longer-term energy-balance regulation taking place through hormones like leptin, sending signals from the adipose tissue, steadying metabolism through waves of energy intake and expenditure.

When body fatness increases in a person, there is an expansion of adipose tissue and a build-up of metabolically active, energy-demanding lean tissue (visceral organs, skeletal muscles, and bones) and a consequent increase in energy expenditure. This leads to increased demand for energy intake to stay in energy balance. Physical activity becomes harder to do, if or when body fatness increases to very high levels, most commonly for mechanical reasons associated with carrying more body weight. Physical activity generally declines with increasing obesity, reducing the dietary energy needed to maintain energy balance per unit of body size. The components of energy balance are also influenced physiologically by changes in each other, defending body energy stores, maintaining energy balance, and preventing shifts in body mass. If energy balance were not controlled by such a system and were responsive only to behavioural mechanisms controlling food intake and volitional energy expenditure, most people would routinely experience wide swings in body weight over short periods of time, which they do not.

One issue with all energy-balance models of metabolism is that none are able to separate cause from effect – or, which came first, chicken or egg. Since obesity can take years to develop in an individual, behavioural and metabolic feedback mechanisms between components of energy balance become increasingly entangled. The developers of an alternative, carbohydrate–insulin, model of obesity claim to have found a way around this chicken-or-egg problem (Chapter 7). The logic runs thus, according to Kevin Hall of the National Institutes of Health in the United States, and his colleagues. Diets high in carbohydrate are particularly fattening because of their ability to elevate insulin secretion. Insulin directs the partitioning of energy toward storage as fat in adipose tissue and away from oxidation by metabolically active lean tissues, resulting in a perceived state of cellular internal starvation. Appetite is increased and metabolism is suppressed, and positive energy balance is promoted, the long-term consequence of which can be obesity. The developers of this model, Hall and colleagues, acknowledge that this model is wrong, along with all other models of obesity, but argue that it is more useful than most, at the present state of knowledge.

So in sum, there are several physiological models of how obesity might develop and be perpetuated, but none of them do it all. Some are suggested to work under specific circumstances; context-specific models can offer explanations as to why some individuals or groups may develop obesity and others not. However, the quest for a universal physiological model of obesity goes on, now increasingly incorporating the brain.

The Gut and the Brain Talk to Each Other

When you go to a party or an all-day buffet, you take your metabolism with you. Your eyes might want to eat every tasty thing on the table, but your brain might get conflicted – "Tastes good, but will it do me good?", or "I'm at a party, does it matter that it doesn't do me good?" I get that conversation too, from the angel on my right shoulder and the devil on my left, both ignoring each other, both trying to convince me to take their path. Pleasure or goodness, which should it be? And how to decide? Well, the way we decide between the pizza and the carrot-stick is more complicated than just a spur-of-the-moment decision. That's because we bring our brain and gut to the party as well.

Obesity, metabolism, and the brain are intricately interconnected, through appetite, eating, satiety and satiation. Your senses add to the mix – you see it, you like it, you eat it. Or not. Then you swallow it, digest it, metabolize it. Or not.

The everyday processes of eating, digesting, and metabolizing we mostly do unthinkingly, but they are regulated physiologically with a system of neural pathways and hormonal mechanisms that involve the brain, the nervous system, the gut, and many of our senses. According to Hans-Rudolf Berthoud and Christopher Morrison of the Pennington Biomedical Research Center at Louisiana State University, the tendency to put on excess body fat can come from any of many malfunctions or lack of adaptation to this system. How do we know what we know about this bodily complexity? Alicia Carriero and colleagues at Purdue University, Indiana, have summarized how thinking has changed since the 1950s, from what they see as being metabolic (1950s to the 1970s), to endocrine (1970s to the 2000s), and to neural (the 2000s to the present-day) eras of obesity.

In the 1950s to the 1970s, appetite was thought to be regulated by macronutrient intake, whether of fat, protein, or carbohydrate. Lipostatic (fat intake), aminostatic (protein intake), and glucostatic (carbohydrate intake) theories of appetite were each set within models where a decrease of one of the nutrients (or metabolite thereof) signalled a bodily need for increased energy intake. In this framing, regulation of dietary intake was largely based on a signal that initiated an eating event, signalled by a physiological need for one or another of these macronutrients. Hunger was seen as the primary driver of appetite and food intake. This model was developed at a simpler time, when obesity and its complexity was yet to emerge as a significant population-level phenomenon. Back then, people mostly would eat at mealtimes with an appetite driven by hunger. According to Jean Mayer, then at Harvard University, physiology best regulates energy balance when energy expenditure pulls appetite along, which it did for most people back then.

Between the 1970s and the 2000s, obesity rates in most wealthy countries rose and accelerated. As physical workloads declined with the increasing mechanization and sedentization of everyday life, food availability and intake increased, along with increasing atomization of eating habits – more people snacked, ate alone, or ate when they wanted to rather than following precise meal patterns, at least in some countries of the Global North. In many countries, many people ate more, usually with larger portion sizes, as food became more commercialized. Across this period, at least in many countries of the Global North, far fewer people ate because they felt hunger, more usually eating because of social and societal cues – because it is lunchtime, for example, or because other people want to eat and you want to join them. This is energy balance as regulated by the push of dietary energy intake, something that Mayer felt the body regulates less well than if driven by hunger. In this period, research focused more on the effects of gut distension from consuming larger amounts at any given time, with increasing emphasis on gut signalling and its influence on appetite and feeding. Many gut hormones were identified across this period that are secreted as nutrients enter the gut, leading to perceptions of satiation. This orientation, towards signals to terminate eating events, was in step with attempts to understand how larger portion sizes could lead to higher energy intakes which could in turn lead to deposition of excess body fat. This primary focus on portion size failed to deliver a solution to obesity, because there are many behavioural ways of getting around this limitation to food intake, especially when someone still feels hungry.

Where the mind goes, the brain goes with it. And so in the 2000s, the science took up with the brain in conversation with the gut. Increased understanding of gut signalling systems, the identification of taste receptors in the gastrointestinal tract (among several other places), and advances in neural imaging techniques all led to a reorientation towards the brain as the central controller of energy intake. The brain had earlier been implicated in both metabolic and endocrine theories of feeding, but not centrally so. By the 2000s, attention had shifted to identifying reward centres in the brain (that were viewed as driving excess food intake) and how they operated. In this neural era of understanding appetite (which we continue to inhabit now), the role of the macronutrients shifted from their contribution to homeostasis to providing signals that promote excessive eating and addictive eating behaviours, with implications for obesity. From this perspective, appetite is regulated in the brain, and the signals for having had enough to eat (by which the desire to eat is quelled) must come from elsewhere in the body. Theoretically, chemosensors anywhere in the body might serve to do this, and to some extent they do, but many have been found in the gut, so much so that the gut has become a key site for investigation of appetite regulation. We know now that gut hormones play a critical role in the regulation of food intake, relaying signals of nutritional and energy status to the central nervous system.

There are models that link energy balance, the endocrinology of the gut, and the brain. Genetics invariably underpin such models, with genetic coding of the enzymes, hormones, and other proteins that do the heavy lifting in metabolism and metabolic signalling being implicated. There are more than 30 hormone genes expressed in the gut, and more than 100 bioactive proteins active in it, making it the largest endocrine organ in the body. It's not just the act of eating though – anticipation of eating, as well as the actual presence of food in the upper gastrointestinal tract, stimulates the release of gut hormones and neurotransmitters from the gut further down. These signals, neurological and hormonal, are involved in both starting an eating event, and the process of eating itself, as well as giving a clue as to when to stop eating. Many of these responses are caused by stomach distension when eating, as well as the biochemical properties of the macronutrients eaten. Eating and metabolism are intricately connected via the gut and the brain, through hunger and appetite, but also (just to make it more complicated) through social cues, and sensory and aesthetic properties of foods, as well as packaging and branding, which are engineered to encourage people to eat beyond satiation. More about this in Chapter 4.

Evolutionarily, the regulation of appetite and food consumption involves adaptations that defend body size and reproductive ability. Nature is full of stresses and insecurities, either immediate or longer-term. Overeating relative to immediate energy needs, overriding the metabolic mechanisms that can maintain homeostasis, is a response to insecurity with deep evolutionary roots (Chapter 5). High reactivity to external cues such as colour, taste, and smell, and subsequent disinhibited eating under conditions of food scarcity, and/or high levels of competition, would have favoured survivorship for our ancestors. Impulsivity – acting without thinking – in relation to food is intuitive.

While I am talking about evolution, let me bring another complication to this system of interrelationships, the microbiota in our gut. This isn't passive but does several jobs. Like marginalizing potentially pathogenic organisms that come into the body as fellow-travellers with food, completing aspects of macronutrient metabolism for the cells of our body, and promoting adaptive immunity and extracting energy from otherwise indigestible dietary carbohydrates (in the distal gut). Each person has slightly different gut microbiota, some of it being inherited from their mother. It is also shaped by what is eaten, what medication is taken, how old a person is, and where they have lived. There is some evidence from University of Alberta researchers that having a furry pet as a child changes the gut microbiota, decreasing the likelihood of developing obesity. We know already that the gut signals to the brain and body through hormones and the nervous system, but the gut microbiota does too, to help us negotiate how we eat, also influencing the cognition and emotion that is linked to eating.

Our microbiota has co-evolved with us, making us less individuals than ecologies. The human body hosts complex microbial communities whose combined membership outnumbers bodily cells by at least a factor of 10. While your gut-microbiota is partly inherited from your mother, there is a core microbiome that most people living in a community share. A part of the gut previously thought to have no function, the appendix, is no longer thought of as being a useless piece of evolutionarily residual tissue, but generates diversity in gut microbiota populations. This includes enrichment of bacteria implicated in insulin regulation. Incidental appendectomy in some forms of obesity surgery influences energy metabolism through changing the microbial balance of the gut. The appendix and its microbiota, hosting mostly beneficial species of gut bacteria, are currently seen as a mediator of homeostasis in the human hosting them. When the gut microbiota is altered by a bout of diarrhoea or other illness (or taking antibiotics), healthy bacteria in the appendix can repopulate it and keep it balanced. In wealthy countries, deviations from the community microbiota are often associated with obesity.

The gut microbiota is also important in programming the hypothalamic–pituitary–adrenal (HPA) axis early in life, and in stress reactivity over the life span. The stress response system is immature at birth and develops throughout the postnatal period, coinciding with intestinal bacterial colonization. Thereafter, gut microbiota influences the development of systems that modulate emotional behaviour and stress, both of which are implicated in comfort eating and overeating to alleviate anxiety and insecurity. In addition, diet quality and gut microbiota work in synergy in effecting affect, or mood. What we eat, therefore, shapes us in far more than a functional nutritional way. Through direct neurophysiological mechanisms, as well as indirect ones via the gut microbiota, food consumption moulds our cognitive and affective being, being intimately connected with experiences of and responses to stress, which in turn influence food consumption and energy metabolism. And in some cases, the development of excess weight.

What Can We Do?

Unlike with a motor car, we can't just switch to a new metabolism when we have had enough of the old one. No, we have what we have, whether it can be likened to a high-performance Ferrari, the Erwin Wurm car, or something in between. While there is some biological variation in energy metabolism in humans – not everyone burns at the same rate – most people can't put obesity down to having a slow metabolism, nor can they attribute being able to avoid putting on weight to a fast metabolism. We can improve the performance of our metabolism, though, so not everything is lost to the lottery of inheritance and genetics. With such an intricate and interconnected physiological system regulating energy metabolism, it might be easy just to give up. But you shouldn't. From a strictly medical perspective, obesity has been described as a chronic relapsing neurological disease requiring lifelong treatment or management. But how can metabolism be managed or treated?

Metabolism is the silent engine that keeps us alive. All the chemical reactions that take place in the body in relation to each other, in cells of the body that convert food into energy and use that energy for running bodily processes, happen within us, mostly without us even noticing. But having a slow metabolism doesn't explain obesity for the vast majority of people. Where it does, it is usually underpinned by genetics that predispose to obesity (more about this in Chapter 2). Different types of energy-balance model of obesity agree with each other in as much as they all frame body weight as being in homeostasis according to levels of food availability and physical activity needed to live life. In societies of abundance, a prudent lifestyle (involving high cognitive control of food intake) is seen as being a precondition for efficient biological control, stable body weight, and maintenance of a set point. This is difficult to do for most people, and weight control advice needs to be nuanced and framed in relation to the metabolism of specific macronutrients and their effects on energy expenditure and appetite.

The market for treating common obesity through metabolism is huge, but research in this area has a long and chequered history. Many drugs designed across the decades to target metabolism have been removed from the market for unintended or undesired consequences – these are well documented. Treatments for monogenic obesity are likely to be much more specialized but perhaps easier to target. One potential form of medication is that of setmelanotide, recently approved by the US Food and Drug Administration for rare monogenic conditions that result in obesity.

White adipose tissue (WAT) can be persuaded to take on some of the properties of BAT, in that genes are switched on that promote uncoupled OXPHOS. Could this work too? Winter swimming seems to have been a thing in the Scandinavian countries since forever, but has become a thing in recent years in the United Kingdom and North America. As well as switching on BAT, cold exposure can naturally induce the beige-ing of WAT, as can physical activity. Could the drying-robe warriors descending upon rivers, lakes, and the ocean in winter be on to something? Adipose tissue both brown and beige can help us burn energy, as both NST and DIT. Win–win. I am sure you want to try this out for yourself, so if you are up for it, take a cold shower now, and don't get out for three minutes. If you survive this, do it every day for a month, and let me know if you get the burn of NST – my email address is in the preface.

But if you can't stand a cold challenge, researchers are looking for pharmaceuticals that can do the same thing but without the pain. That might work better for people with obesity, who are better insulated against the cold, and thus have enhanced body heat retention and also lower BAT responsiveness to the cold. Anything that reduces the efficiency of making chemical energy from food energy should help, in this age of plentiful calories.

At the individual level, most dieting and weight-loss approaches to obtaining and maintaining healthy weight make use of one form of energy-balance model or another, with logic based in metabolism. They don't seem to work so well across longer time frames, giving only modest weight loss for either exercise or dietary restriction, with only slightly greater weight losses when exercise is combined with dietary restriction. This has led many researchers to challenge the usefulness of energy-balance models as the basis for weight-loss interventions, because interventions that reduce body fat stores without dealing with physiological compensatory responses that promote the recovery of lost fat are more likely to fail than those that do. Giles Yeo views weight loss to be much less about calories than about food, and much less about overall fat intake than about the type of fat you eat. More about this in Chapter 4. Long-term success of weight reduction based on energy-balance models may only be possible when dietary restriction and physical activity are engaged in fastidiously, with strong cognitive restraint against overeating. Meta-analyses of multiple weight-loss trial studies have shown that most types of intervention can produce weight loss in the first six months, but beyond that, it's tricky. Interventions involving diet-only, or diet plus exercise, or pharmaceuticals plus diet produce weight loss that is sustainable beyond a year, but this requires strong reinforcement not to overeat. If you can climb this metabolic mountain of negative energy balance and weight loss, the chances are that you may be able to remain at lower body weight across many years. But unlike climbing Mount Everest, it takes two years or more to climb Mount Metabolism. And even then, about a third of dieters don't adapt to lower levels of energy intake, but instead gain weight after dieting because of a mix of reduced energy expenditure, increased consumption of calories from fat, decreased dietary restraint, increased hunger, dietary disinhibition, and binge eating. More of this, and what you can do, in Chapter 7.

From an evolutionary perspective, raised post-dieting appetite, increased food consumption, and weight gain are adaptations that defend body size. This evolved in times when obtaining enough food was a real day-to-day challenge, which it is no longer. We retain this set of adaptations while not being able to rev-up the metabolic motor to a degree that can compensate for all the additional calories we are now able to consume. The drugs we have had up to now haven't seemed to help a huge amount, but there is the current promise of semaglutide, about which more is said in Chapter 7. So, putting metabolism to one side, we turn in the next chapter to the purveyors of cheap calories, the food industry. And to the modern-world food environments that predispose us to obesity.

4 I Blame the Food Corporations

Corporate Logic

"Look, if it's not my genes, it must be the environment?" I overheard someone say this in a pub. Well, yes and no. One of the visible aspects of urban environments – and let's face it, most of us are urban now – is food. Ever-present junk food, aisles of frozen pizza and snack foods in the supermarkets. In the United Kingdom, which built much of its colonial power on the triangle of relationships among industrialization, slavery and plantation production, sugar is historically a huge industry, and you can see sugar-based products in stores everywhere. It hurts people's lives through dental decay, obesity, and type 2 diabetes. In the United States, perfectly edible maize is systematically turned into high-fructose corn syrup, a substance that is even more damaging to health than sugar.

Epidemiologically, the food environment is conceptualized in terms of physical access to food resources – especially supermarkets, grocery stores, fast food restaurants, and convenience stores. If you can't purposefully (yet) turn off genetics associated with obesity, then maybe you can do something about the food environment. In this chapter I work through the idea of an obesity-causing food environment, and the idea that food choices are to blame for our own body fatness, dispelling the misunderstanding that it is somehow simple and monolithic. Rather, it is complex, layered, and interactive. Those environments have not been constructed explicitly to cause obesity; nobody wants that, for sure. But the food system, which is one very important contributor to this environment, was initially designed in the US in the early twentieth century to ensure food security through the production of cheap calories, an idea that spread throughout the world especially with the work of the Food and Agriculture Organization of the United Nations.

The term 'obesogenic environment' is widespread and used to characterize environments that encourage eating too many calories and not getting enough physical activity. Most descriptions of such environments refer to very particular structures and geographies, usually involving urbanism. While urbanism is certainly part of the story, the fact is that the current rise in obesity in the world is happening mostly in rural places. And even if we acknowledge that urbanism was probably associated with the greatest rise in obesity up until the past couple of decades, urban environments do not automatically predispose to obesity. Genetics and epigenetics are important (Chapter 2), the latter especially so in relation to undernutrition and exposure to some toxic metals in early life, but linking the idea of obesogenic environment to urbanism is messy. This is particularly so in relation to food, since food supply in urban places can differ hugely, reflecting assemblages of urban design and use, past and present. As we now understand urban places a little better, planners and policymakers across the world are finding ways of improving the environments in which we live to make them healthier, less 'obesogenic'. Towns and cities change, and they might actually be becoming healthier for us now. So, to start at the base, what is an environment, and why is it important to know this, in relation to obesity?

Of Environments and Individualism

In obesity research, the boundaries that, for example, separate the individual from nature and the normal from the pathological stem from a period in Western nineteenth-century Romanticism when the term 'environment' was coined to make separations, or dualisms, in nature. In earlier centuries, Rationalist thinkers, beginning with René Descartes, had already defined a formal separation of the mind of the body in order for religion and science to co-exist: religion could concern itself with the mind, ceding dominion over the body to medical science. This gave rise to a kind of dualist thinking that separated the individual ('man') from their body, and later, from their environment. The term 'environment' was framed by Scottish writer Thomas Carlyle in 1828, at a time when industrialization was tearing up both nature and the small-scale human societies within it, largely replacing them with technology and turning farmers into industrial workers. In this framework, individuals began to be conceived as largely separate from their environments – as masters, planners, and interlopers – rather than organisms who were at the mercy of the environment. Individualism thus grew as capitalism and urban places grew.

The non-Western world did not necessarily conceive of such dualisms, or held other ways of thinking about humans in the environment. Colonialism and globalization brought Western ways of thinking to the non-West, so that today much of the thinking concerning obesogenic environments is infused with Western bias.

Prior to the mid-2000s, obesity research and intervention dealt with environments in a dualistic way, relating the measured experience or state of the body (via the body mass index, BMI, for example) to measured factors outside the body (access to fast-food restaurants, for example). This led to considerable knowledge of dualistic relationships, which, while individually valid, contributed to a cacophony in obesity-related research output and in policymaking. In the early 2000s, there were attempts to 'de-individualize' obesity research and intervention. Tim Lang and Geof Rayner, of City University London, attempted to do this using an ecological framing, by analysing how an interconnection of factors since the 1960s led to the emergence of population obesity and its related chronic disease issues. The UK Government think-tank Foresight attempted to do something similar for obesity policymaking by using a complexity framing that alluded to the interaction of many factors tipping populations to obesity (Figure 4.1). These attempts at de-individualization acknowledged the need to ultimately remove dualisms from obesity research to make it tractable for policy, and to bring it in line with twenty-first-century political thinking.

These approaches did not gain traction, largely because individualism has remained a very powerful force in current neoliberal society. Not surprising, then, that organizations involved in obesity policy and prevention have struggled to move away from individualist framings. Despite excess body fatness being recognized by many as being an outcome of ecological processes or of complexity, finding ways of making these ideas tractable for policy and for

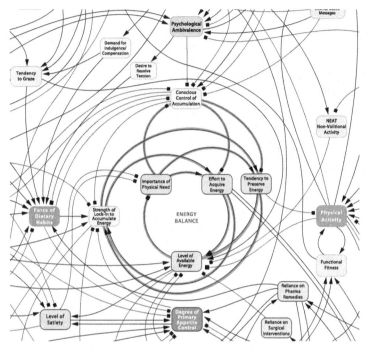

Figure 4.1   Inner core of the Foresight Obesity Systems Map.

making interventions within existing political frameworks has proved very difficult indeed.

In this context, the idea of environment as something 'out there' beyond the body continues to be widely accepted in obesity studies and intervention. While it is accepted that interactions of factors can lead to obesity, what are most usually studied are relationships between people and things, where things include food.

The research literature on obesity and environment mostly assumes the environment to be acting on the individual body and not the social or political one, and does not usually reflect the interactive nature of obesity production. Furthermore, the situating of food within the obesogenic environments framing most often sees the rise in obesity rates as being rooted in ways of life as they relate to food, planting the unit of analysis firmly at the individual level, when the formulation, production, delivery and cost of foods, all influential in what people actually eat on a daily basis, is largely in the hands of corporations.

Obesogenic Environments

At one level, the idea of environmental backgrounds that predispose to obesity is easily understood; it includes all aspects of environments, physical and social, that promote gaining weight, and that are not conducive to weight loss. In this framing, obesogenic environments are easily identified by their having a great preponderance of motorized transport and of sedentary occupations, and the cheap and easy availability of high-fat, high-refined-carbohydrate foods (so-called ultra-processed foods). In general, what makes life convenient and energy efficient at the individual level can also promote obesity. Obesogenic environments can be found across the urban landscape of most wealthy countries, but it was in Australia that the idea was given intellectual form. The concept, and the analytical framework with which it was described, were developed by public health researchers there in the late 1990s in response to an identified need for methods that would allow the environment – which was increasingly being acknowledged as a contributor to population-level obesity – to be rigorously and systematically studied.

Obesogenic environments have not always been with us. In many cities in the US, Europe, and Australia, modernist metropolitan plans were developed on the ground from the 1950s onwards, based on low-density suburban housing, car transport, and freeway systems, with supermarket-based food shopping as part of this assemblage. The growth of obesogenic environments was helped on its way by steady displacement of small local shops that could be walked or cycled to. Modern cities structured around separated land use, with work in one place, and shopping, recreation, and sleeping in other locations, promoted car use and with it a displacement of daily food shopping by shopping on a larger scale less often, with often less healthy food being bought and eaten. Systems of fast-food retail set close by major highways and often in or near gas stations allowed the growth of eating on the go, displacing more structured eating patterns within the household. In Copenhagen, a city that has resisted becoming obesogenic from the start, there are, to the present-day, very few large supermarkets, even though the world's very first food super-market was opened in this city and continues to thrive. Most supermarkets in Copenhagen are small, limiting food choices with a nudge toward healthier eating. People walk, cycle, or use public transport to get to them, so people buy less on any visit, reducing the space to buy and take home unhealthy food relative to healthier food. If you don't have the convenience of the motor car, you are limited in how much you can carry home in one go. Fewer supermar-kets and fast-food outlets are set close by major highways because few people have cars at all in this city, the public transport system (including walk-ways and cycle paths) making cars much less of a necessity than in most wealthy countries. In most other wealthy countries, obesogenic environments have emerged and grown, with ever-increasing commuting times and the speeding up of everyday life such that cooking (and eating together) becomes difficult, even for those heavily committed to the idea. So how did we get here?

According to Barry Popkin, of the University of North Carolina, urbanization, westernization, and economic change across the second half of the twentieth century resulted in major shifts of diets across the world toward lower nutrient density and higher energy density. Alongside this, obesity emerged firstly among wealthier sectors of society and then in higher proportions among poorer sectors. This is Popkin's 'grand narrative' of nutrition transition, which, as grand narratives go, is not bad at describing the past, especially with respect to relationships between nutrition and disease, infectious and chronic. It is, however, implicitly colonial in framing, sitting uneasily in the decolonizing present day. Nutrition transition continues to be the framing used in public health whenever links between newly affluent populations and dietary change are under view. In relation to obesity, there is an implication that the emergence of obesity in the Global South has been different from its emergence in the Global North – as an outcome of population exposure to obesogenic environments in wealthy countries, but an outcome of economic modernization in poorer ones.

If anything, though, the difference in obesity production between Global North and Global South is a matter of time and scale. Modernization of the Global North began over 500 years ago. The Global South has seen modernization only in the past several decades. This, along with the decline in food prices in a global food system that prioritizes calories and open markets, has helped to drive the rapid emergence and expansion of obesity everywhere. In the Global North, modernity has also involved the expansion of cities requiring motorized transport (more about this in Chapter 8), increasing economic inequality, and growing availability of cheap ultra-processed food (UPFs), all of which have contributed to obesity. Add to this mix new and more efficient marketing and distribution infrastructures, extended and modernized roads and ports, greater access to foreign suppliers and food imports, globalization of food consumption patterns, and the spread of obesity across the Global South is clearly part of the same phenomenon as observed in the Global North. These food system changes have resulted in a shift towards great availability of food energy, notably refined carbohydrates (including sugar), and of fats and oils, which have been linked to rising population obesity.

The 'modern' obesogenic environment can probably be traced back to the ways in which colonialism shaped the food systems of the colonized. In East and South Asia, and former communist states in Eastern Europe as well as in countries of Africa, the trajectories of rising obesity are in part outcomes of global, historical, and colonial processes. Food and agriculture have been central to many colonial projects of 'civilizing' local populations across the Global South, setting the context for subsequent dietary change with post–World War II modernity. The westernization of diet in post-colonial settings follows the dietary changes that took place during colonial domination, and the creation of new markets for fats, oils, refined carbohydrates, and UPFs more generally. The opening up of local and national markets to global food has happened differently in different countries, and across different time-frames. In China, this took place after the major economic transformation of 1985, whereas in Brazil and Mexico, markets opened up to global food in 1974 and 1988, respectively. In the Cook Islands, where I carried out research in 1995, dramatic changes in diet, declining physical activity, increasing body size, and rising obesity rates began in 1945, following colonially driven diet change by the British from 1881, when many good eating habits of the population were displaced by bad ones in relation to health outcomes. In the next section, I examine how what has come to be called 'the food environment' by epidemiologists is linked to obesity.

Obesity and the Food Environment

Shauna Downs, of Rutgers University, and her colleagues have developed a typology of food environments, which gives some background to usage of this term in obesity research and intervention. Used in ecology to refer to food chains of different species and their abundance and nutritional quality, the term 'food environment' was appropriated in the 1970s for describing human food supply systems. This incorporated food-related practices in institutional settings such as schools and workplaces, as well as built environments and neighbourhoods within them. Since then, the food environments construct has been increasingly applied to relationships between food, diets, and chronic disease in wealthy countries, increasingly using systems-based socioecological models to examine food availability and choice. In the current neoliberal world, where choice is a politically charged idea and where people have increasingly come to be characterized as consumers, the food environments construct now incorporates consumer choice, as food systems are seen to structure the availability, affordability, convenience, and desirability of foods.

In public health, the food environment is usually reduced to the physical presence of food through proximity to food store locations, the distribution of food stores, food service, and any physical entity by which food may be obtained, or any connected system that allows access to food. Conceptualized in terms of physical access to food resources – especially supermarkets, grocery stores, fast food restaurants, and convenience stores – this approach defines food as a physical exposure or risk factor. For example, food outlets, or more broadly, places where people are exposed to (the wrong types of) food, are often reduced to 'exposures of interest' in relation to where people live, which can then be quantified as forms of poor diet, and statistically analysed in relation to body weight or BMI.

A cultural bias in this work, largely because most research of this type has been carried out in the US, is that it sees supermarket access as providing healthy food options, which is not universally the case. The exposures approach implicitly accepts that health risk is also embedded in the consumption of certain types of food, as in the case of foods high in saturated fat and risk of cardiovascular disease. This was initially formalized in terms of healthy (or unhealthy) food composition, the absence (or presence) of toxins in food, and subsequently the extent and nature of industrial processing. Heitor Paula Neto, of the Federal University of Rio de Janeiro, has argued that in addition, many food additives can influence weight gain via immune system mediated metabolic dysregulation. The exposures approach doesn't overtly consider the forces that mediate purchase and consumption of food such as product placement, marketing, and branding. Nor does it consider sensory cues that might stimulate people to overeat. Deborah Cohen, of the Rand Corporation, Santa Monica, California, sees the ubiquitous exposure to food and the omni-presence of food advertising to be an external stimulus for feelings of hunger and overconsumption.

Alternatively, Christopher Turner, of the London School of Hygiene and Tropical Medicine, and his colleagues, frame food environments in relation to nutrition and health without excluding bias created by assuming that supermar-kets provide healthier choices. They see the food environment as comprising external and personal domains. The external domain refers to factors influen-cing food acquisition and consumption that are not directly influenced or controlled by individuals. This is seen as having four components: food avail-ability in stores; food prices; characteristics of food products and food vendors available; and broader marketing and regulation environments. The personal domain includes factors more directly related to individual agency, again with four components: physical access to food; affordability; convenience; and individual preference, taste, and knowledge. Health risk in relation to food is therefore layered, with macro-level factors more under political economic control hovering above individual-level factors. This framing helps to clarify who should do what in terms of intervention against provision and consumption of obesity-risky foods.

The impact of the World-Wide Web on food choice and consumption – beyond corporate marketing and promotion – should not be overlooked. The food environment is now also shaped by the digital world in the almost universal use of just-in-time computer-algorithm-based expert systems in food supply chains. There are also forms of buying and selling food products and services through digital technology which change the characteristics of food vendors, especially with online grocery shopping and food delivery services using websites or smartphone apps. Sarah Bates and her colleagues at the University of Sydney see these developments as matters for concern for public health. In relation to nutritional quality of food offerings made available by digital food service outlet platforms, the promotion, availability, and accessibility of unhealthy food choices is very high. The association of such foods with diet-related chronic disease is much higher when compared with meals prepared at home. Jeremy Brice of the University of Oxford has studied food-related digital marketplaces in the UK and found them to broadly fall into two categories – curated and non-curated. At the high end, the logic of choice in the curated digital food marketplace is to provide high-quality goods and vendors with food quality or service standards that are above the legal minimum. At the low end, digital marketplaces attempt to capture as many as possible of the vendors and consumers active in that market, setting no standards above the legal minimum, and open to any vendor not legally prohibited from trading. This is a poorly regulated market, at least in the UK. A voluntary approach through curation, offering consumers good food choices, however defined, is emerging, in this regulatory 'wild west', where you can buy what you want, as much as you want, and eat it, away from social scrutiny. It might not be a recipe for disaster, but it might be one for growing obesity.

Research carried out by Melina Mejova, of the ISI institute in Turin, and her colleagues has shown that with the changing sociality that has come with Web 2.0 since 2004, obesity is now more strongly linked to social interactions over food posting on social media than with fast-food restaurant prevalence, at least in the US. They also found that web-based social approval favours the consumption of unhealthy foods, especially those high in sugar. Online activities shape other factors linked to obesity in addition to eating behaviours, including bodily dissatisfaction and physical activity patterns. With all this emphasis on food and healthy eating, it is important to identify which foods are actually complicit in the production of obesity and chronic disease, and this is what I turn to next.

Food, Eating, and Obesity

Part of the creation of modern food environments is the classification of foods into different types, and according to epidemiological risk. In wealthy countries, such typologies have been internalized by most people. This is evident with everyday usages of terms like 'gluten-free', 'vegetarian', 'vegan', 'low fat', 'free from', in characterizing the types of diet we might eat. Thinking of food as a risk exposure is very much in line with sociologist Ulrich Beck's framing of risk society, in which most risks in modern society are reflexive and self-induced, in contrast to earlier times. We might eat vegan because we see it as reducing our personal risk of developing chronic disease. But we might see it as reducing risk of environmental degradation, or poor animal welfare, or climate change. The risk category of UPF has had most attention recently in relation to obesity. But can you really recognize an ultra-processed food when you see it?

I like a good definition, as does Michael Gibney of University College Dublin. He has observed the changing definitions of UPFs since Carlos Montiero, of Sao Paolo University, first defined them in 2009. Montiero published a food classification scheme, NOVA, based on the degree of processing of foods, of which UPFs are the most extremely processed. Table 4.1 shows some of the

2009	Extracts from whole foods with no, or small amounts of minimally processed foods added, plus salt, other preservatives, and cosmetic additives.
2010	Mixes of processed culinary or food industry ingredients with unprocessed or minimally processed foods.
2012	Formulated from ingredients typically containing no whole foods, not recognizable as versions of existing foods. Most ingredients not available separately to consumers, majority of which are additives, including bulkers, sweeteners, sensory enhancers, flavours, and colours.
2014	Formulated from substances derived from foods, containing little or no whole foods. Durable, convenient, accessible, highly palatable, often habit-forming, usually not recognizable as versions of existing foods, but may imitate the appearance, shape, and sensory qualities of existing foods. Many ingredients not available to consumers separately, some

Table 4.1   (cont.)

	directly derived from foods, such as oils, fats, flours, starches, and sugar, some obtained by further processing of food constituents. Majority of ingredients include preservatives; stabilizers, emulsifiers, solvents, binders, bulkers; sweeteners, sensory enhancers, colours, flavours, and processing aids. Micronutrients may be added. Processes include hydrogenation, hydrolysis; extruding, moulding, reshaping; preprocessing by frying or baking.
2015	Industrial products made entirely or mostly from substances extracted from food (oils, fats, sugar, starch, proteins), derived from food constituents (hydrogenated fats, modified starches), or synthesized from organic materials such as oil and coal (colourants, flavourings, flavour enhancers, and additives for attractive sensory properties).
2016a	Industrial formulations with ingredients often including sugar, oils, fats, salt, antioxidants, stabilizers, and preservatives. Can include substances not commonly used in culinary preparations and additives which imitate sensory qualities of unprocessed or minimally processed foods or culinary preparations of them, or to disguise undesirable sensory qualities.
2016b	Formulations of ingredients that, besides salt, sugar, oils, and fats, include food substances not used in culinary preparations, especially flavours, colours, sweeteners, emulsifiers, and additives used to imitate sensory qualities of unprocessed or minimally processed foods or culinary preparations of them, or to disguise undesirable sensory qualities.
2017	Industrial formulations containing some mix of salt, sugar, oils, and fats, and food substances not commonly used in culinary preparations, including hydrolysed protein, modified starches, hydrogenated or inter-esterified oils, and additives used to imitate sensory qualities of unprocessed or minimally processed foods or culinary preparations of them, or to disguise undesirable sensory qualities.

Modified from 2019 work by Michael Gibney.

Table 4.1   Evolution of definitions of the term 'ultra-processed food' (2010–2017)

changing definitions of UPFs between 2009 and 2017. The first definition alludes mainly to the use of both food additives and salt in food products, while the second introduces the putative impact of UPFs on accessibility, convenience, and palatability. Subsequent definitions become more detailed, including more elements and building on previous definitions. The definitions have been further enriched by the inclusion of foods containing ingredients that are not available to the general public, foods made overwhelmingly with food additives, foods that are extensively fortified, foods synthesized in a laboratory, and foods based on organic materials such as oil- and coal-based additives and flavouring compounds. There is continued emphasis on the inclusion in foods of high levels of salt, sugars, and fats, as a starting point for their definition as UPFs. According to a review carried out by Leonie Elizabeth at Deakin University, Geelong, and colleagues, UPFs are associated with the following disease category groupings: obesity and cardio-metabolic risk; cancer, type 2 diabetes and cardiovascular diseases; irritable bowel syndrome; depression; and frailty conditions. They are also linked to all-cause mortality. There is no evidence of any positive health benefits of UPFs beyond their being safe from bacterial and other contamination.

Michael Gibney has catalogued the categories of foods that fall into the UPF pit, and this is summarized in Table 4.2. Some foods are categorized as being ultra-processed, regardless of which definition is used, notably foods high in fat, high in sugar and refined carbohydrates. If you have the time and energy, you could take Table 4.2 with you into a supermarket, and you could tick off just how many items are UPF. The list given in the table won't help you, though, if you easily succumb to your evolutionarily based eating instincts.

Doughnuts, as deep-fried pastries, fall into the 2010 UPF category. Just think about standing in front of a doughnut stand right now, trying to choose one to eat, any type you like. It is sweet, fatty, sugary, each bite offering a sensory experience, coating the mouth with sweetness while chewing and swallowing. Another bite almost automatically follows the first one, repeating the magic moment when the sugar hits the taste buds and signals pleasure to the brain (Chapter 3). The refined carbohydrate and fat in the doughnut do not satisfy hunger quickly though, so it is easy to eat another one. Think about doughnuts in general and their diverse world, made with a variety of fillings, favours, toppings, sprinkles, designed to speak to our evolutionarily based

| | Year | | | | | | | |
	2009	2010	2012	2014	2015	2016a	2016b	2017
Cereal-based products	Breads; breakfast cereals; cereal bars	Breads; breakfast cereals with added sugar; cereal bars	Sweetened breads and buns; bread and other cereal products; breakfast cereals, 'energy'/ 'cereal' bars	Breads, buns; breakfast cereals	Sliced bread, hamburger or hot dog processed bread; sweet breads; cereal bars	Breads and baked goods which include hydrogenated vegetable fat, whey, emulsifiers, and other additives; morning cereals, cereal bars	Mass produced breads and buns; breakfast cereals	Mass-produced packaged breads and buns; breakfast cereals, 'cereal' and 'energy' bars
Cakes & pastries	Cookies (biscuits)	Cakes & pastries; biscuits (cookies)	Cookies (biscuits); pastries, cakes and cake mixes; desserts	Cookies (biscuits); pastries, cakes & cake mixes; desserts	Sweet and savoury biscuits	Cake mixes	Cookies (biscuits); pastries, cakes and cake mixes; desserts	Cookies, pastries, cakes, and cake mixes
Sweets & confectionery	Chocolates, candies and sweets	Chocolates; confectionery (candies)	Chocolates; candies (confectionery)	Chocolates; candies (confectionery)	Processed sweets and treats in general (candies, ice creams, chocolates)	Confectionery; sugar substitutes and sweeteners, and all syrups (excluding 100% maple syrup)	Chocolates; candies (confectionery)	Chocolates; candies

Jams & preserves	Snacks	Dairy products & substitutes
Jams (preserves)	Chips (crisps); savoury and sweet snacks	Ice cream
Preserves (jams)	Chips (crisps); savoury and sweet snacks	Cheeses; ice cream
Preserves (jams)	Chips (crisps); many other types of sweet, fatty or salty snack products	Ice-cream; margarines and spreads; fruit yoghurts
	Chips (crisps); sweet, fatty or salty snack products; energy bars	Ice cream; margarines
	Chip-like snacks	Margarine
	Packaged snacks	Not listed
	Sweet or savoury packaged snacks; cereal and energy bars	Margarine and spreads
	Sweet or savoury packaged snacks	Ice cream; margarines and spreads; 'fruit' yoghurts

Modified from 2019 work by Michael Gibney.

Table 4.2 Classification of ultra-processed foods

desire for food novelty. Have you ever heard a doughnut speak? I think I have; they don't seem have much vocabulary, merely whispering repeatedly, "Eat me". Before we knew about food ingredients, sweet taste gave our ancestors some signal of the energy content of any particular food. It is no accident that we feel pleasure when consuming calories – we have an evolutionary drive to seek them out. The doughnut is engineered to deliver the maximum amount of pleasure, an energy bomb, a very slow-acting weapon of mass destruction, contributing its share of the obesity-producing food payload. In addition, UPFs contain additives, some of which, as obesogens, may contribute independently to weight gain. The doughnut is complicit in making people put on body fat, as are so many of the UPFs, however they are defined. But it's not just about the food we eat, it's about how we eat it, which is what I turn to next.

In Western society, we eat, as the Japanese would say, when we are not hungry but when our mouth is lonely – 'Kuchi sabi shii'. Or because we can practise urban foraging very easily, filling up with food, eating on the go. Eating on the go means that you are not giving the food you are eating the appreciation it deserves. With UPFs, we eat more for pleasure and other reasons, like 'It's lunch time,' rather than to appease hunger. In Japan, eating on the go is frowned upon, people seeing it as plain poor manners to walk or do other things while eating. The use of digital technologies also promotes unhungry eating. It is easy to overeat when eating while doing something else – distraction eating, it has been called. Still in Japan, there is a saying, 'Hara hachi bu', which means eating until you are not quite full. Eating at a set mealtime when hungry, avoiding snacking, practising hara hachi bu, people can avoid overeating, and thereby also avoid gaining excess weight. I know that things are changing in Japan, that these practices are challenged by many, and that obesity rates are rising, but all of these changes are taking place from a very low baseline. Obesity in Japan is around one-tenth of that in the US. People practising Hinduism see food as being sacred, most of them eating vegetarian diets. Viewed from this perspective, there is something deeply indecent about growing cattle for slaughter, as in the Western world, but not only that, grinding down the lower-quality meat into burger material, to be consumed unthinkingly, quickly, and on the go. When we eat slowly, with foods that are much less calorific than doughnuts, we can match satiety to satiation. But we can easily overshoot this with foods high in fat and sugar.

And overshooting with calories day by day, month by month, year by year, we build up body fat and contribute to the globally rising tide of obesity. Eating in a slow and appreciative manner, stopping before you are full, helps resist weight gain.

Eating without thinking is easy in the food environments of most wealthy countries. Eating beyond bodily physiological signals to stop, eating at random times and places, eating to quell negative emotions and affect, eating for comfort. Social and evaluative stress, anxiety, and worrying about how other people respond to you or see you, are some factors among many that can contribute to obesity via poor dietary choices. Living in stressful circumstances contributes to poor dietary choice, especially where there is so much poor food (in terms of nutritional quality) to choose from.

Gorging on food in a disinhibited way when food is widely available is an evolutionarily adaptive mechanism for dealing with one of the most fundamental of insecurities, that of food. It is only in recent decades, with improved food security in wealthy countries and the emergence of obesity at the population level, that it has become maladaptive. Distraction feeding is another form of eating without thinking, while reading, driving, watching a screen, easily leading to overeating. Popcorn and the movies go together in many people's minds, but this is a particular form of distraction feeding. I see people with headphones all around me these days. Some are talking to people as they go, others are listening to podcasts (educational ones, I choose to think) or music. Eating while wearing a sonic device, as well as using electronic devices during mealtimes, also influences what people eat, usually towards UPFs.

What Can We Do?

It's out of your control – that's the first thing to say. The food environment continues to change, and research into its relationship with obesity is like tracking a moving target. So what can we do to ensure healthy, non-obesogenic eating, in this ever-changing landscape? Support for individuals is key – with the latest food environment knowledge, and strategies for being able to negotiate the food environment. Otherwise, we are just rabbits staring into the headlights of an oncoming truck filled with UPFs on its way to restock the stores and supermarkets. Better framing of food environments in relation to nutrition and health can help.

At the population level, the vagueness of the concept of obesogenic environments has made it attractive to policymakers because they can interpret it in different ways and according to different ethical principles. People live in environments that are constructed through social, political, and economic processes, and this is reflected in food policy and provision. What has become obesogenic is often a matter of chance – no individual, agency, corporation, or institution planned for obesity. But governments tend to show the seriousness with which they take obesity through population measurement, classification, and reporting. This ensures that concerns about obesity (as a measurable outcome) are incorporated into the regulation of systems – food, urban planning – that are considered to produce it.

An intervention that is proving effective against the future development of obesity is sugar taxation. Increasing the price of products containing sugar alters consumption, while increasing the price of sugar-sweetened beverages (SSBs) reduces the price gap between them and healthier but often more expensive drinks. Taxes on SSBs have become a health policy of choice because of the strong link of drinking these substances to obesity, their lack of nutritional quality, and their high price elasticity. SSB consumption is very high across the world, being the biggest source of added sugar in the diet of people in the US. Unlike eating foods, there are no compensatory mechanisms after drinking beverages to induce satiation, so you are likely to just keep drinking them, piling on empty calories.

Making sugar and its products more expensive reduces sales, but maybe you could go a step or two further, and try to purge your diet of sugar. In 1972, John Yudkin, of Queen Elizabeth College, University of London, wrote a book called *Pure, White and Deadly*. It wasn't about cocaine, but in some ways it might have been. Animal studies show that behaviours associated with eating sugar and with drugs of addiction overlap with each other. These include bingeing, craving, tolerance, withdrawal, cross-sensitization, cross-tolerance, cross-dependence, reward, and opioid effects – is this list long enough for you? There are also overlaps in brain neurochemistry with use of drugs of abuse and sugar, at least from animal studies. You wouldn't put cocaine on your cornflakes, so why would you do so with sugar? But because of these effects (granted they are weaker with sugar than with drugs of dependence), it is difficult to just give up. Ways of quelling the demands of our evolutionarily programmed sweet tooth include withdrawal and desensitization, or displacement with real foods. Michael Goran and Emily Ventura, of the University of Southern California, have put a lot of thought and energy into both of these, offering ways of retraining the palate and adjusting the diet to go without sugar.

To make real change, we can't expect people to just change their eating behaviours with sheer willpower. Instead, we need to find ways to make our food systems better. Tanya Schneider, of the University of St Gallen, and colleagues have researched digital food activism – groups of digitally connected people striving to do exactly that. What else can you as an individual do? You can strive to eat healthily – the science behind eating fruit and veg for health will never put a rocket into orbit, but it saves lives here on Earth. There are many microscale projects doing this now, across the world. A challenge is to scale these up to a degree that food corporations stop pushing UPFs and respond by producing and selling real food. Across recent decades, there has been a chase to the bottom in terms of producing cheap calories, by producers and retailers. We all deserve better than this.

5   I Blame Society

A Social Disease

In wealthy countries, the least well-off put on the most weight, as do people who are constantly under stress. Put them together, stress and under-privilege, and you have the makings of an imperfect storm, differently made in different contexts – just add ultra-processed food (UPF). Which is cheap, easily available in most places, and a significant contributor to obesity-causing food environments. Can't you blame society, really? Before you can think about addressing this question, it is first important to have some idea of what society is. At base, a society is a group of people who are socially connected in some way, and/or occupy the same social or geographical space, usually bathing in the same political and cultural water. Social status matters, and this influences their behaviour, including in ways that can influence their body weight. If what I eat is shaped by what other people eat, because we regularly eat together (as with family) or because we as friends share common interests that extend to our eating patterns, then this aspect of society might influence the likelihood (or not) of me putting on excess weight. At a more macro-level, society, through institutions and government, structures what people can and can't do, and this influences their behaviours through laws and taxation, for example. But people have the ability to act in their best interests, however they frame them, and to some extent resist dominant political and institutional laws and edicts when they are not in their best interests. So if society contributes to the production of obesity, is it a 'social disease'? The song 'Gee, Officer Krupke', in Leonard Bernstein's musical *West Side Story*, parodies the concept of cumulative risk in response to multiple stressors, by tunefully unpacking juvenile delinquency as a social disease. Societal structures, through low income, poor education, and low socioeconomic status, as well as precarity and insecurity, are the most common multiple stressors in the construction of obesity as a 'disease of society'. These stressors, how they operate and interact, is what I describe in this chapter, as well as examining how individualism in present-day society relates to these and other stresses in the production of obesity in everyday life.

Obesity in Society

When we read media accounts of how levels of obesity are changing, almost always rising, the natural unit of reporting is that of the nation-state – the UK, the US, Australia, and so on. Breaking the numbers down within countries, there are widespread inequalities in obesity as well as inequalities in income, occupation and education which influence the development of obesity in different but overlapping ways. As a generality, obesity is more common among the poor in wealthy countries, and among the rich in poorer ones. In wealthy countries, obesity used to be more common among wealthier people prior to the 1960s.

In an international comparison, Lindsay McLaren, of the University of Calgary, has shown that more educated people in wealthy countries are less likely to carry excess weight than less educated people. She showed that it's different for income, though, wealthier women being less likely to carry excess than poorer women, wealthier men being more likely to. Men usually don't think too much about their body weight, but if they do, it's because a brush with chronic disease has pushed them to do so. Weight management takes time and resources, as does eating healthily. Women generally have higher cultural beauty ideals than men, and if men of high socioeconomic status (SES) have few concerns about their body image, they may also be more relaxed about consuming UPFs and gaining weight.

Income, occupation, and education only partially reflect women's status in society, there being other forms of capital (sociologist Pierre Bourdieu identified three major forms of capital: economic; social; and cultural. Figure 5.1

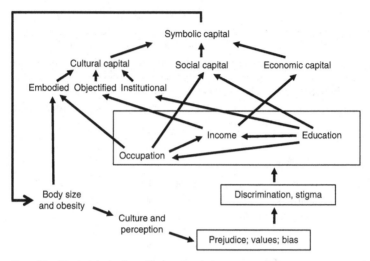

Figure 5.1   Obesity, the body and forms of capital.

shows the relationships among these and other related forms of capital, and obesity). Economic capital is the easiest to understand – money talks. If you want to eat healthier food, higher income is not a prerequisite, but it helps. Social capital is distinct from SES and represents group cohesion and cooperative behaviour for mutual benefit. In everyday life, women rely much more on social networks for psychological and physical support than men. Having greater social capital ameliorates stress and is associated with lower body fatness. Cultural capital overlaps with economic capital, and represents a person's assets, including education, ways of dressing and talking, that place them in society. Its relationship with obesity is in respect of social signalling and network effects – in wealthy countries, the higher placed someone is, the less value body fatness has, and the more likely they are to associate with other people who place low value body on body fatness. Institutional cultural capital consists of recognition of individuals by the state (most usually in terms of academic credentials, qualifications and honours) or by working in a prestigious organization. It overlaps with education as a form of status, but it can further discriminate on the basis of the status of different educational institutions.

In addition to economic, social, and cultural capital, embodied capital reflects bodily properties that are either consciously acquired or inherited, such as beauty, bodily symmetry, poise, and athleticism. American supermodel Cameron Russell is, according to the blurb for the Ted Talk she gave in 2012, 'Tall, pretty, and an underwear model . . .'. She openly acknowledges having won 'a genetic lottery' in relation to her embodied capital, as well as having graduated from Columbia University. She is well placed in society with her 'beauty bonus', the economic benefits, and the education that it has brought. Usain Bolt, now retired from athletics, is considered to be the greatest sprinter of all time. I saw him win gold in the sprint relay at the London 2012 Olympic Games, breaking a world record. The whole stadium would have loved to have been Usain Bolt that glorious warm summer night. Many women would love to have Cameron Russell's physical attributes. Sadly, most of us normal people can neither be Russell nor Bolt. Money, economic capital, might help us acquire and maintain some of these bodily properties, but it is not a prerequisite. Given the differences in cultural valuation of body size among different groups and populations, obesity carries higher value as embodied cultural capital in groups that value greater body weight than among those that do not. In Kuwait, Saudi Arabia, and the United Arab Emirates, for example, such cultural valuation has not diminished as economic prosperity in these countries has risen.

Yet another form of capital is objectified capital. This represents the value of relationships between people and objects that confer status upon them. It can include prestigious brands of foods and designer-labelled clothes, as well as more traditional measures of social position that can be obtained through living in the right neighbourhood, living in an expensive house, and the consumption of high-status foods (which varies across societies). While economic capital can help in buying objectified capital, it is not a requirement. For example, objectified capital can be attained through consuming branded fast foods among those who have little economic capital, such fast food being a potential contributor to obesity among those of low SES.

Returning to Cameron Russell, we can think about how these different forms of capital can be aggregated. She has spread her portfolio across different forms of capital – embodied, economic, educational, symbolic, institutional. In wealthy countries, slimness is a form of embodied capital that is sought by many women. Media and literature representations in Western societies have largely privileged the slender female body for over a century. Idealized images of women in mass media also privilege thinness and are among the most powerful influences on how women view themselves. Social media have only amplified and added power to these persuaders. In the UK, people of higher SES are more concerned about body shape and engage in more efforts to lose weight than people of low SES, but overall, women show more weight concern than men do, regardless of SES. Compliance with thin bodily ideals is a way for women to signal their appropriateness for prestigious employment and to find reproductive partners of high quality (should they want them). In evolutionary terms, fatness, within bounds, is advantageous, but in societies where controlled reproduction predominates (as in most wealthy countries), it has low value as embodied capital. Women bear the burden of negative factors that go with having obesity, like stigma, blame, and fat-shame (more about this and the stigma associated with racism and social class in Chapter 6). Women can also biologically transmit, through reproductive and early-life history experiences, factors that influence the likelihood of their children, should they have them, of developing excess body fatness. Women's status in relation to obesity differs in in some important ways to men, with occupational status being often much less important than appropriate embodiment.

Obesity is higher among many marginalized groups in wealthy countries – among population minorities and Indigenous populations, among those with mental illness and military veterans, for example. Inequalities in population obesity include a mix of genetic and epigenetic factors (Chapter 2), metabolism (Chapter 3), access to cheap UPFs (Chapter 4), and poor access to physical activity resources when living in poor or dangerous neighbourhoods (Chapter 8). If you are poor, consuming UPFs can relieve stress and anxiety, especially if you have low social capital and live a wealthy country where individualism is king or queen, and where obesity has the strong look of a social disease. Individualism can isolate people, and this is another aspect of obesity inequality, which is considered next.

Individualism and Obesity

It is a story that we are all familiar with – the hollowing out of society. At school we are told we can be anything we want to be, and that we are all individuals striving to meet our potential in life. The reality, when entering adult life, is less enchanting – only a small number of people can truly become what they have sought to be. Most people have to lower their expectations of life, while learning to function in a world of changing norms and low levels of social support, especially in many wealthy countries. Individualism has roots in the Global North which are several centuries deep, but it has only become important to the obesity story in the past four decades or so, with the growth of consumerism and of neoliberalism. In combination, both of these, as socioeconomic and political forces, have created more fluid notions of society, with a hollowed-out shared public domain, and have, in many places, overwhelmed territorial identities and eroded often solid social identities based on the workplace.

Neoliberalism is a political model that transfers control of economic factors from the public sector to the private one and opens markets to trade. This ideology took hold in some wealthy countries from the 1980s, with increased economic integration and deregulation of trade and capital flows across the world. Increasingly, many more countries now practise some form of market liberalism, including countries with emerging economies, like China, Brazil, and India. Integration of trade has greatly contributed to economic growth, and globalization has enhanced the economies of many countries, but the greatest increases in obesity rates are in the world's regions that bought into these processes earliest. The worldwide proliferation of transnational corporations (transnational food companies among them) that has accompanied globalization may have played a key role in influencing rising rates of obesity, especially through the marketing and sale of UPFs, soft drinks, and fast food from the 1980s onwards (Chapter 7).

Is it stressful to live life the neoliberal way? You bet, especially if you are at the bottom of the tree and the squirrels at the top are not dropping enough nuts down for you to survive. Individualist ways of living involve constant self-evaluation, and this can be challenging – the bottom line is always that if you fail, you only have yourself to blame. All this, in an environmental and structural world where you are constantly being persuaded to make the choices that are best for capitalism but often the worst for you. Ted Schrecker and Claire Bambra, of Durham University, have argued that we currently live in an age of neoliberal epidemics, where the labour market and the world of work is insecure, and where physiological responses to insecurity predispose to obesity and ill-health. An overriding value placed on individualism in market-liberal societies, described as neoliberal selfhood by Stephen Vassallo, of American University in Washington DC, may be a driving force for obesity. Neoliberal selfhood emerged as a dominant mode of being in many Western societies in the 1980s with the rise of Thatcherism and Reaganism. Margaret Thatcher's market liberal agenda was, in her own words, a programme of change in which 'The method is economic but the object is to change the soul.' This coincided with the acceleration of obesity rates in the UK and the US. Neoliberal selfhood is now well-embedded in most Western societies and has several notable characteristics that predispose to constant self-evaluative and social stress. For example, the neoliberal self tries to make rational choices and is organized around an ethic of efficiency and productivity, while knowing it is impossible to be an economically rational agent all of the time. The neoliberal self takes responsibility for its own life outcomes – if things go wrong, there is no-one to blame but one's (neoliberal) self. The neoliberal self strategically manages choices and ceaselessly pursues the increase in personal value, making everyday life instrumental to the extreme. Unsurprisingly, it assigns especial value to selfhood, making for constant self-evaluation and self-monitoring. More than a generation since its emergence, neoliberal selfhood has become linked to low self-esteem, increased anxiety, isolation, and selfishness. Neoliberal selfhood allows certain freedoms, but creates pressures and stresses. Social and evaluative stresses engage the hypothalamic–pituitary–adrenal (HPA) axis most, and a likely mechanism linking neoliberal selfhood to the development of obesity is dysregulated appetite and stress-related eating. Amy McLennan of the Australian National University and I have shown that neoliberal framings of public health locate the natural unit of obesity policy and intervention at the level of the individual.

Neoliberalism has undermined personal stability and security to a greater degree among people of lower SES. In the US, commercialism and consumerism have grown at the expense of political participation, and shrinking civil society has contributed to the fragmentation of social life. In the UK, from the time of the Margaret Thatcher administration (1979 to 1990), governments of all ideologies have framed policies overwhelmingly around the construct of the individual consumer as a target for regulation. This formulation of consumer citizenship means that individuals are not merely to be free to choose, but to be obliged to be free, and to understand and enact their lives in terms of choice. The conflict embedded in this idea is that political theory defines citizens as being willing to serve the common good while consumers are defined by their individualist 'pleasure-seeking' characteristics. Along with cheap energy-dense food (Chapter 4), the rise of neoliberalism and individualism across most societies has linked good citizenship to individual consumption, including that of food. What you consume and how you consume matter, and not just to you, but to the government.

For a person with obesity, individualism can be a curse, since the easiest fallback position on obesity – for governments and in everyday life – is that of personal responsibility. In this framing people with obesity become their own victims and only have themselves to blame for the suffering and blame they experience. More about this in Chapter 6. Media representations of obesity often individualize it while taking a fatalistic position in relation to its reversibility, with genetic attributions and explanations making this worse (Chapter 2). In the US, individualism and obesity are used as a means of discussing themes society is uncomfortable with, such as poverty, race, and/ or ethnicity. Individualism, like obesity, brings stress and insecurity, especially in relation to employment contracts, and in the US, to health insurance. And in the absence of social support, insecurity and anxiety are assuaged often with the cheapest and most available drugs on the market, which are sugar and UPFs.

Stress and Insecurity

While inequalities in obesity can be measured epidemiologically through the categories of gender, ethnicity, income, education, and occupation, the relationships between obesity and insecurity are trickier to show scientifically, but are nonetheless real. So how does insecurity differ from inequality? Taking an example from economics, while economic inequality is the variation between people or populations in their incomes and assets, economic insecurity is the uncertainty of having an income and of assets persisting into the future. Such insecurity is ameliorated by the likelihood of continued employment, and the availability of welfare provision, savings, and pensions. Other forms of insecurity include those of health provision when ill, and having skills that are marketable and transferable into the future. An analysis of obesity rates across wealthy nations shows the extent of social welfare to be a powerful correlate of obesity. I very much like the Nordic countries and their approaches to obesity, which are largely about preventing its development in the first place. They have among the very lowest obesity rates of all wealthy countries. Work carried out at the University of Oxford by Avner Offer, Rachel Pechey, and myself has shown that adult obesity rates in Nordic countries are lower than in English-speaking neoliberal nations, but do not differ from those in continental European family- and community-oriented nations, like France and Italy. What do the Nordic countries have in common with family-oriented European countries? Both of them value a communitarian approach to life above an individualist one, although they have very different ways of doing it. Nordic social democracies, which place sociality central to politics, are nearly a century old, while continental European models of society run much deeper, and place the community at the core of political life. In contrast, countries practising neoliberalism place the individual at the core of politics, with more limited or eroded communitarian and community-level values. Non-standard parental work schedules (working at weekends, at night or during evenings) have also been shown to be associated with childhood overweight and obesity, possibly because of increased stress that comes with disrupted family life. Insecurity from illness (as expressed by private medical expenses as a percentage of disposable income, a proxy for risk of incurring private medical costs) has the strongest relationship with obesity among all individual measures of social insecurity. This is because of the high costs of healthcare in countries like the US, where falling ill is a given (as in all societies), while the individual ability to accommodate the financial burden of healthcare is not. In the US, data from the Survey of Economic Risk Perceptions and Insecurity analysed by Yale University's Jacob Hacker and his colleagues show that insecurity, whether expressed as worry or as economic shock (such as unemployment, or runaway economic inflation), is far greater for households with limited education and with lower income than in households with higher income and education levels. An exception to this is wealth shock, where, for example, a drop in value of retirement investments or home foreclosure affects the wealthier and the poorer, the less and the more educated. In the study of Hacker and colleagues, worry is much more stratified by SES than any aspect of economic shock, suggesting that the psychosocial stress of everyday life that associates with weight gain and obesity is likely to be mediated through inequality.

At the individual level, insecurity and inequality influence the production of obesity through stress alleviation by comfort eating and binge eating. Anxiety about body weight can be deeply personal, but also play out in social contexts, there being clear links between directly experienced social inequality, anxiety, and dietary energy intake. An experiment carried out by Boyka Bratanova of St Andrews University, and an international team of researchers, has shown that people whom they experimentally induced to view themselves as being poor (as opposed to being wealthy) ate more dietary energy than those who viewed themselves as being wealthy. They also showed that people who had previously experienced inequality (viewing themselves as being either poorer or wealthier within the same social grouping) were more anxious than those who saw themselves as being equal in such contexts. Bratanova and colleagues also showed that such anxiety leads to greater energy intake among experimental subjects who have a strong need to belong to a group. The implications of this are stark – the effects of inequality and insecurity on obesity-related behaviours are tightly bound together, through social processes.

Stress and anxiety can recruit overeating as an alleviation response, especially when energy-dense foods are cheap to buy. Putting on weight is a biological response to insecurity (Chapter 4). Humans are highly responsive to external food cues such as colour, taste, and smell, and in times of stress, disinhibited eating under conditions of food scarcity and/or high levels of competition would have favoured survival for those most likely to eat in a disinhibited way until fairly recent times. These days, the stresses of everyday life are different from those on the African savannah around a million years ago or so, but we are still that animal with the same evolved mechanisms for dealing with stress. These mechanisms are common to all mammals and involve engaging the mesolimbic dopamine reward system of the brain, which rewards survivorship activities, like eating and sexual intercourse, with pleasure. The foods that give the most pleasure are especially those high in sugars and other refined carbohydrates. In modern life, wandering around a town or city, it is difficult to avoid contact with such foods and their often brightly coloured attractive labels. And if not the foods themselves, then the advertising for them – fast food outlet hoardings, street and shop advertising, advertising on the Internet, people posting their best experiences with UPFs, programmes in media about foods and eating, sometimes on demand as with mukhbang, often about eating far too much. These abundantly present everyday food cues are easy to respond to in the context of the stresses and psychological insecurities of everyday modern life we all experience.

It gets worse, though. Have you ever thought about eating that doughnut from Chapter 4? The one that appeals to your inner childhood self? And then you eat it and it's gone and you are full of regret? Well, human impulsivity to eat especially tasty things is normal from an evolutionary perspective, especially if it is situational and related to pleasure, sociality, and distraction. Sometimes you just want to eat and eat, even though you know you shouldn't and you know you are not hungry – you want to eat and eat because you have had a stressful day, because your partner dumped you, because your boss took a dump on you – all of these reasons and then some more. Some psychologists call it binge eating, an evolutionarily based physiological feeding adaptation to food uncertainty, which doesn't need a hunger stimulus from the gut, especially when very tasty foods are on offer. Some other psychologists call it hedonic hunger, eating for pleasure, when the hunger you are assuaging is a hunger for happiness. The mechanism of hedonic hunger has been deliberately hijacked by food corporations whose business is to trade in highly palatable, energy-dense foods. More about this in Chapter 7. In the meantime, what's a woman or a man to do?

What Can We Do?

It takes society, not individuals, to create social and economic inequality, and inequalities in obesity rates. If obesity is one outcome of living in an unequal society, then we have only brought it on ourselves, especially across the past four decades, with the rise and normalization of neoliberalism and the neo-liberal self. Consumption and citizenship have become inextricably linked since the 1990s, before which they were located in opposing private and public domains, and associated with competing inner- and outer-regarding norms and actions. Inequality is not going away anytime soon, and politically, people have been reduced to units of consumption, regardless of whether they are rich or poor. Half a century ago, Jean Baudrillard, of the Paris Nanterre University, had anticipated the importance of consumption in society by saying that, in the same way that medieval society was balanced on God and the Devil, so modern society is balanced on consumption and its denunciation. The rhetoric of choice has penetrated most aspects of policy formulation and implementation since the 1980s, and obesity has not been exempt from this. Governments often use models of rational choice in constructing obesity as an economics issue, but then use the rhetoric of choice in models for obesity regulation. Both rational choice and the rhetoric of choice have individualism at their centres. The latter is used discursively in framing individual freedoms and agency, while rational choice assumes that individuals will serve their own interests in giving them the most benefit in the decisions they make in life. The trouble is, human beings are never fully free from influence, nor rational in their behaviours. In recent times, the rhetoric of choice has been employed by governments in their use of nudge tactics to frame how people should make decisions in everyday life, while recognizing that food corporations also employ the rhetoric of choice often in quite different ways, when marketing and branding their products. With respect to obesity, governments may nudge us toward healthy eating choices, while food corporations push us to make their products, often unhealthy ones, our choices, usually with the blessing of the same governments.

A placard in a charity shop window in Oxford reads 'Make poverty history'. If only it were that easy. Could doing away with inequality be easier than doing away with poverty? Actually, in the dominant political climate of our time, it is much harder than doing away with poverty, if not impossible. Inequality is built into capitalism – it needs it to function. Obesity is one of the damaged tiles on the floor of economic progress, which doesn't get fixed because the person on maintenance doesn't have tile cement for obesity. At the moment no-one does, but we can hope that semaglutide (Chapter 7) will help.

So what happens is worse than a broken tile. People with obesity are blamed for the damage done by the consumerist way we are all encouraged to live. While we can't topple capitalism (much bigger forces than you and I have tried and failed), we can at least acknowledge the damage it does, as well as the good it can create – which, in relation to obesity, is to engage economists to model the likely outcomes for obesity of different kinds of policy approach, in the hope that the worst effects on excess body fatness might be mitigated. To some extent this was done in the UK in the landmark Foresight Obesities policy process, where the idea of obesity as an outcome of societal and biological complexity was first given serious consideration. Four policy scenarios were floated, as summarized in Figure 5.2. Linking any of these to future outcomes in terms of obesity rates and obesity inequality shows that some policy approaches are more likely to be successful than others (Table 5.1). I had lunch with a doctoral student at my Oxford College recently, and in an animated conversation she summarized what I was thinking in one breath – 'Inequality isn't inevitable, it's a policy choice.' Incorporating obesity data (such as collected in many countries now) into

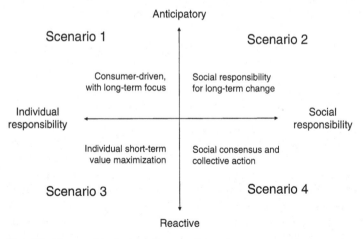

Figure 5.2   Four possible obesity policy scenarios.

		Policy scenario			
		S1	**S2**	**S3**	**S4**
Impact	Population	Increase	Decrease	Increase	Decrease
	Socioeconomic	Little or no change	Decrease	Increase	Decrease
	Childhood	Decrease	Decrease	Increase	Increase

Modified from Butland et al. (2007).

Table 5.1 Likely impacts on obesity rates relative to United Kingdom rates in early 2000s, according to four policy scenarios

econometric modelling would make it much more transparent that obesity is not inevitable, it's a policy choice.

At the national level, governments can regulate environments and food systems, and through taxation and social support can influence the extent of inequality in a nation. But the political economic systems that especially favour neoliberalism have helped create obesogenic environments (think Conservatism in the UK, Republicanism in the US), and have helped make cheap UPFs an attractive drug of choice among many seeking solace from the stresses of everyday life. Obesity policy, in neoliberal society, has perhaps unsurprisingly continued to place emphasis on the individual and much less emphasis on societal approaches. In a systematic review of intervention types at the individual, community, and societal level for reducing socioeconomic inequalities in childhood obesity, Claire Bambra of Durham University and her colleagues found that at best, most interventions do not increase inequalities in rates of obesity, but nor do they reduce them. While seemingly impossible to shift, inequalities in obesity rates are neither ahistorical nor politically neutral. Public health may assume a level policy playing field for obesity intervention, but this is never the case. Upstream structural interventions by politicians have the potential to reduce obesogenic influences, but organizations that have a keen interest in the structure of such interventions include corporations, the world views of which are governed by profit and not welfare. Sharon Friel, of the Australian National University, and her colleagues have shown how corporate power can influence inequalities in obesity through trade agreements, in that industry representatives greatly outnumber representatives from public interest groups, giving an imbalance between the goals of trade and of consumer protection. Through their keen involvement in such regulatory activities, corporations help design the structures that influence food and health in favour of their interests rather than the public good.

Gøsta Esping-Andersen, of the Universitat Pompeu Fabra, Barcelona, has called for more child-centred social investment strategies by governments, as life chances, including health, depend increasingly on the cultural, social, and cognitive capital that citizens can amass. Following this, Michael Marmot and colleagues at University College London have offered two policy goals that could help to reduce inequalities in obesity rates. These are to create societies that maximize individual and community potential, and to ensure that policies are centred on social justice, health, and sustainability, rather than with economic gains in mind.

Usually using the rhetoric of choice, advertising, government, and media try in different ways to persuade us that we can truly shape our individual identities and our personal destinies. Applying the rhetoric of choice to what and how we choose to eat may seem like an act of free will, until you think about what is shaping our choices. While we can't really have it all, we can strive to live within our physical, economic, and cognitive means. We can try to evaluate the messaging – is it really helping? And to be critical of the idea of choice – what is constraining my ability to control my body weight, if I am urged to consume according to my choices (which are usually the choices of others much more powerful than me)?

We can try to live less stressful lives – easier said than done, though. Or we can find ways of reducing stress that do not involve eating or any self-harming practice (like smoking, drinking alcohol, or using illicit drugs). Physical activity, whatever that might involve, works for lots of people. But even there, the physical structure of where you live might preclude exercise – you might live in suburbia with very limited public transport, or you might live a very urban life where the surroundings are physically dangerous or serve very poorly for physical activity. More about this in Chapter 8. Being critical of how life is shaped for you, rather than by you, is a good first step to working out just how much control of your circumstances you can actually have. Paraphrasing Bob Dylan's 'All Along the Watchtower' (some of you may know the Jimi Hendrix cover of the song), 'There must be some way out of here, said the joker to the thief' – words that are evocative of individual powerlessness. Obesity for some is one outcome of such powerlessness. Often fixing one thing, even something seemingly unrelated to obesity, can help with weight control, especially if that one thing fixed reduces insecurity and uncertainty. There are always choices we can make, but we have to be aware of the choice architecture (and who built that choice architecture) if we are to choose well.

6 You've Only Got Yourself to Blame

Don't Put Me Down

I go to the swimming pool and everybody's body is on show, including my own. I don't have rippling pecs, and I am in my 60s, an age when you think I wouldn't care about my body anymore, but I do. Another swimmer, in her 30s, is just getting out of the water. She is 'a big girl', and gets looks, of the wrong kind, even though I have watched her plough the lanes and work hard, keeping enough stamina back to sprint her final lap. If I am self-conscious of my body, how self-conscious is she? Every look is a dagger to her self-esteem. I try to put myself in her place, chanting to myself, 'Don't put me down, don't put me down.' People who say, 'You've got yourself to blame' have got it wrong. Even though the evidence is that body stigma only contributes to obesity, people stigmatize large body size – especially in the Global North among poorer people, females, and Black and Indigenous peoples. I discuss how obesity stigma comes from the type of moralizing thought that is embedded in present-day Western societies. I go on to consider how obesity stigma is used to develop and maintain social hierarchies in times of food-plenty.

Why Do People Pass Judgement on Other People's Bodies?

Moral judgement is rife in everyday life, and we often judge actions as good or bad without knowing much about the context in which those actions have been made. We do much the same with people. The world moves fast and is constantly changing, and we often need to make judgements about situations as they unfold in short, often instantaneous real time. Obesity unfolds in real time too – extended time. Obesity is seen by many as an outcome of acts undertaken in shorter, even instantaneous, real time, before your eyes, morally judged as bad. We can't dismiss these acts of moral judgement – as Frank Furedi, of the University of Kent, has written, moral judgement is central to moral responsibility and is therefore central to the maintenance of moral boundaries. The sum total of millions of moral judgements, people showing approval or imposing moral sanction, keeps society straight without recourse to the heavy cosh of the law. In general, this isn't a bad thing, but should it be so in relation to other people's bodies? It certainly seems to matter to a lot of people, but before applying moral sanction to other people's bodies, shouldn't we consider why it matters to society as a whole?

When it comes to food, physical activity, and displaying the body, is it right to evaluate actions attached to moving, eating, and bodily display, to ascribe motives for doing them and to characterize them as good or bad, as right or wrong, as beneficial or harmful, as virtuous or vicious? What does the obese body and its actions in the world do to threaten the social order, or the worlds of others? We judge people's bodies all the time, and ascribe virtues and sins according to what we see and how we value what we see. What underpins snap-judgements of all kinds, and what we do with those judgements, is fundamental to how society runs, and speaks volumes about our anxieties about our own bodies, our own eating patterns, and our own movement behaviours. So let's start unpacking it.

It all starts with beauty (Chapter 5), which is in the eye of the beholder and therefore difficult to subject to scientific scrutiny. I was having a casual conversation about what I do for a living with Alan, an engineer. Once he knew I did research into obesity, there was no stopping him. He was very soon lecturing me about obesity, and the fact that this was not his area of expertise while it was mine did not put him off his stride. 'In many parts of the world, people find fat bodies beautiful', he offered as a final answer as to why obesity is a huge issue outside of the Western world. Yes but. In many parts of the world people find body fatness attractive – there is a lot of evidence to support that view – and this may contribute to rising obesity in a changing world where ultra-processed foods (UPFs) are widespread. Larger body size has been seen as attractive and indicative of attributes such as health, fertility, beauty, wealth, and power, in many countries in the past, including those of the

West, and in many countries of the Global South until quite recently. In a cross-cultural comparison of body size norms in different societies in the Global South including Nauru, the Cook Islands, Samoa, and Malaysia, most people have until recently favoured a level of body fatness above the now-international, body mass index (BMI) norm of health. African American women have generally preferred body size that is larger, on average, than European American women, while African American women classified as overweight and obese perceive themselves as being healthier, more attractive, and more attractive to the opposite sex than White women of similar weight and age. There have also been groups in Africa and the Pacific Islands where some form of ritual fattening used to be practised, to promote fertility and marriageability, and where large body size was a form of embodied capital. Most such societies now have rising and often extremely high levels of obesity.

Sociocultural factors, such as participation in the global economy and exposure to Western ideas, has shifted body image perceptions worldwide. Many communities and societies in which obesity has risen in recent decades and that previously desired and/or accepted larger and fatter bodies have come to prefer thinner bodies. This is the case for African American women, Turkish adolescents, Pacific Islanders, the Ojibway-Cree in Canada, urban Native American youth, and Korean children. The desire for thinner body size is increasing in many countries, even if attaining a thin body against a backdrop of globally increasing body fatness is now more an aspiration than a reality for most. Although high cultural valuation of body fatness might have contributed to the emergence of obesity in many countries, it might cease to be an important contributor for future generations. The idea that beauty is a final and concluding explanation (as Alan, in my conversation with him, felt it was) worries me, because it takes us to a dangerous place we are all aware of. I call it Stigma-Land. In Stigma-Land, everyone judges everyone else – for the size of their house, living in the wrong neighbourhood, and if not that, then living on the wrong side of the street of the right neighbourhood. There is always something to judge people on, in Stigma-Land. It can also be wearing the wrong things, having the wrong haircut, being too short, and, of course, being too fat. Maybe you already live in Stigma-Land; for sure, the village I live in can sometimes feel like Stigma-Land.

Stigma and Obesity

You know it when you are on the wrong end of stigma. Negative comments, looks, or general demeanour, things to put you in your place. In its broadest sense, stigma describes *negative attitudes or discrimination against someone on the basis of something, be it a disability, disfigurement, mental health trait, or other bodily aspect.* You can see how open to stigmatization obesity is, when a fat body is there for all to see. It takes two to dance the stigma dance, one to dominate and another who doesn't want to be there at all – the stigmatizer and the stigmatized. It is a deeply disturbing form of moral judgement, which in respect of obesity has very little to do with the direct health consequences of excess body fatness. Stigma can be openly inflicted but also subtly so, like a clip to the ankle of a soccer player who then tumbles to the ground. Like many perpetrators of a soccer ankle-clip, the stigmatizer says, "Who me?" when challenged. They get away with it so often, when in my view they should be red-carded, shamed off the field. Women are much more likely to experience weight stigma than men, as are poorer people compared to wealthier people, and Black people compared to White people, in all kinds of settings and contexts, especially in the Global North. Weight stigma is a deeply cultural, moral, and social process, linked to stress. It is widely practised, often in institutional settings, including medical clinics, at the workplace, as well as in media representations. It accompanies the weighing and quantification of fat bodies that is a precondition to the framing of obesity as medical, economic, or public health problems. The stigma that surrounds body fatness and obesity in most wealthy countries often creates social disadvantages in employment, education, healthcare, and interpersonal relationships.

In the Global North, the pursuit of thinness and bodily perfection among women contributes to the pathologization and stigmatization of body fatness. In the US, body fatness and obesity have been stigmatized for over a hundred years. There, women are 16 times more likely than men to report weight-related employment discrimination, while women with obesity are much less likely than thin women to hold down high-paying jobs, even after accounting for socioeconomic differences. Obesity drags down women in another way too – it hinders their social and economic mobility more than it does for men.

More generally, people with lower intergenerational economic mobility are more likely to carry excess weight in adolescence, regardless of country-wide level of economic inequality. While weight bias is common in most wealthy countries, it is increasingly so in economically emerging nations. It translates into inequalities in employment and healthcare, often due to widespread negative stereotypes about persons with obesity.

In formal media, obesity is represented as an irreversible problem. A recent headline in a leading UK online newspaper starts with "Little Britain? Fat Chance!" The *Mail Online* was reporting on new projections of future obesity rates. This might seem fairly innocuous, but formal media also find ways to individualize excess weight, through stories like this one I just invented, based on a true account I read by journalist Lizzie Wingfield:

> I went to the doctor having lost a lot of weight, nearly twenty kilograms – a lot of weight. I was expecting her to be amazed by how much I had lost, how much better I looked, but no. I guess that my doctor sees a lot of people every day and that she couldn't recall my body size the last time I saw her, but it feels truly awful when you realise that you are only one of many little rocks by the side of the water.

Not only is the journalist, Lizzie Wingfield, not the only little rock by the side of the water, she, the little rock, is looked at and examined by non-medical others who pass moral judgement. Weight stigma is manifested in stereotypes, rejection, and prejudice toward her, and all the other little rocks by the water. One of the most common ways of expressing weight stigma is through verbal attack or verbal bullying. Saying things that attack someone's sense of self, with a clear intent of inflicting psychological pain, devalues and humiliates the person on the receiving end. That is just in-person everyday life. Social media has expanded this dramatically. A study carried out by Wen-Ying Sylvia Chou of the US National Institutes of Health and her colleagues, analysing around 1.4 million posts from a range of social media channels including Twitter, Facebook, Flickr, and YouTube, found that over 90 per cent of them link obesity to negative, misogynist, or derogatory terms. Furthermore, Janet Tomiyama of the University of California, Los Angeles, has linked weight-based aggressive comments to negative mental health outcomes, including depression and anxiety, in people with obesity. Online activities shape eating behaviours as well as bodily dissatisfaction, and it is easy to see how online stigma can easily beget such negative outcomes. Yongwoog Andrew Jeon, of Northern Illinois University, and his colleagues analysed the content of YouTube comments that discuss overweight individuals or groups from two videos that went viral – 'Fat Girl Tinder Date' and 'Fat Guy Tinder Date'. Overweight women in these videos were much more commonly attacked verbally by men than by women, while overweight men were not attacked so much, by either women or men.

According to Alex Brewis (Slade), of Arizona State University, there are four interrelated ways in which stigma can lead to excess body weight and obesity. First, if fat stigma negatively affects people's exercise, diet, and health-seeking behaviours (Chapters 7 and 8), then this can lead to weight gain or impede weight loss. Second, weight stigma is usually associated with a physiological response to psychosocial stress which promotes appetite and weight gain. Third, stigma can lead to weight gain through changing social networks, if it leads to people associating with each other according to body weight, physical activity norms, and/or habitual dietary intakes. For example, Nicholas Christakis and James Fowler, both then of Harvard University, showed a large sample of US citizens in a social network to cluster according to body weight. The fourth mechanism linking stigma to body fatness is through softening the psychological effects of discrimination by seeking out comfort foods that are usually ultra-processed. Intergenerational weight gain or weight retention can operate through these mechanisms, via stress, insecurity, and/or low SES. In the US, obesity stigma is an enormous issue, producing social disadvantages in employment, education, healthcare, and interpersonal relationships.

Is there an evolutionary basis for weight stigma? Wen-Ying Sylvia Chou thinks so. Starting with verbal aggression – men are more likely to stigmatize women with unforgiveable words than women are men. Evolutionary psychologists claim that in the deep past, males would have attempted to maximize their reproductive success (that is, to have as many offspring as possible) by inferring a potential mate's reproductive success from physical appearance, much more so than would have females, who would have primarily sought mates with high resource acquisition properties, such as possession of territory, industriousness, and high social status. According to Chou, such differences have shaped patterns of verbal aggression, to the present day. A man may be verbally attacked for lacking ambition, resourceful skills, or money, while a woman is more likely to be attacked for being physically unattractive. However, this may be mediated by societal norms, especially where a high proportion of women are in the work force, where many women reject traditional 'house and home' expectations of them, and where the traditional male–female gender binary is increasingly questioned. The meaning of 'physically unattractive' changes across the generations and varies from society to society. Excess body weight was extremely unusual and difficult to achieve among ancestral humans, and it might well have been an aspect of beauty. These days it is the other way around, with the lean and fit body forming a Western ideal of female beauty. Fatness may have been associated with fertility in past populations, but in the present context of controlled reproduction, it no longer carries such value for women.

Moralizing Thoughts Don't Lead to Virtuous Actions

Sometimes people think they are doing a good thing by showing their concern about an issue – climate disasters, death, disease, the fate of others when facing tragedy. These are all issues individuals can get behind and signal their virtue to others, either face to face or on social media. Take a look on your social media, and see how common it is for people to signal goodness in some way. Just focusing on this makes it look like the world we know is going through an epidemic of goodness. In the physical world, it isn't like that. People seem happy to broadcast their high moral standing without doing much to actually make the world a better place. Virtue signallers on social media enjoy the privilege of feeling better about themselves by doing very little, according to journalist James Bartholomew. Virtue signalling often consists of completely costless actions, but signals to others that the signaller is a good person, which has the pay-off of (online) friendship and social status. Humans evolved a sense of morality because people who convince others of their moral qualities reap strong social benefits, even reproductive benefits. How could a virtue signaller make the world a better place for people with obesity? It depends on how honest the signal is. Across human evolution, the ability to discriminate a true ally from a false friend could have had life-or-death consequences. We are left with a residue of this when we scan for moral hypocrisy, or when someone publicly endorses a moral standard but behaves in violation of it. The evolutionarily based tendency to scan the horizon for false virtue signalling is particularly strong among people who see themselves as carrying excess weight. According to Lee Monaghan, of the University of Limerick, we have gone through decades of moral panic about obesity, and this has consolidated the notion of excess weight as being morally repugnant, unhealthy, and socially irremediable.

Men's understandings of their own body weight are connected to the ways they display their moral worth, and include how heaviness, healthiness, and physical fitness are not seen as being incompatible, and resisting standardization by relative weight criteria like the BMI (Chapter 1). Men are therefore judged differently from women and are less likely to be objects of virtue signalling, with all its ambiguities. According to Virginia Chang, of the University of Pennsylvania, and Nicholas Christakis, 32 per cent of men in a sample of US males classified as overweight by BMI criteria think that their weight is about right; only 11 per cent of overweight women in this sample feel the same way. In the same study, 38 per cent of women of normal weight by the same criteria think themselves to be overweight, while only 10 per cent of men do. Since there is a strong association between self-perceived weight status and weight control behaviour, usually independently of objective weight status, women are especially sensitive to both weight-based stigma and potentially ambiguous virtue signalling.

Virtue signalling is also something that people carrying excess weight may practise themselves, especially when in the role of 'Being a Good Fatty'. Feminist writer and activist Kitty Stryker has written about this in her blog 'Everyday Feminism'. She describes the ways in which she has learned to be a Good Fatty herself, in her words, the fat person who can never be socially acceptable, but who publicly flogs herself for the sin of carrying excess weight. She sees The Good Fatty as coming in many guises, especially the performative, apologetic, trying-not-to-be-fat Good Fatty. The Good Fatty acknowledges and accepts the othering of themselves, both in their personal and professional lives. Othering involves some individuals or groups being defined and labelled as not fitting into the norms of a dominant social group. It influences how people perceive and treat those who are viewed as being part of an in-group (us) as against those who are seen as being part of an out-group (the others). The Good Fatty must show competence in front of the medical profession and in the world of work, as well as in public everyday life. The Good Fatty is the person with excess weight that people in the normal range of weight will tolerate, and the role involves survival strategies. According to Stryker, the six main ways that a person of excess weight can survive moral judgement in the wider world of thinner people are as follows. Firstly, Good Fatties exercise, despite the fact that the gym and the pool are common sites of fat shaming. Secondly, Good Fatties eat right. Just knowing this, people with obesity often don't eat in front of other people or will go hungry in order to look 'good' eating the 'right' foods. Eating in hiding is a way to avoid the food police, that is, people who judge anyone on what they eat based on to their body weight. This extends to food shopping – what person carrying excess body weight can enjoy food shopping when they know other people's eyes are on them and their shopping trolleys, judging what they buy? Thirdly, Good Fatties go on weight-loss diets, often feeling pushed to try new diets in order to show that they are 'behaving', even if that diet isn't necessarily the healthiest for them. Weight-restriction diets can actually contribute to weight gain as well as loss in confidence if a diet fails and impulsive eating results in a rebound of weight. Fourthly, the Good Fatty has to dress impeccably, because to do otherwise invites the moral judgement of being sloppy as well as fat. Sweatpants and tee shirt in public? That doesn't cut it, not even on a casual Saturday morning off work. Then there is the challenge of finding good clothes to wear, as well as the money with which to buy them – affordable clothes that fit and flatter a larger body can be expensive. Overweight men might get away with dressing down, but overweight women, no, never. Most men don't have to worry about make-up either, something that is critically important for women carrying excess weight, to present a good face to a weight-critical world. A fifth way to be a Good Fatty is to not show too much skin. The body fat police notice when women of excess weight show some thigh/arm/belly/cleavage. This extends to social media, where women of excess weight posting a little flesh get threats and negative comments. People of excess weight may engage more commonly with forums and communities that are defined through bodily identity. Sarah-Rose Marcus, of Rutgers University, has shown that people with excess weight engage more with fat acceptance sites through hashtags related to positivity and self-love than with neutral or negative social media signals. Members of online fat acceptance communities distinguish against outsiders by attempting to reframe beauty, and provide support by complimenting users' appearances and providing information and resources on how to maintain a good body image at higher body weight. Finally, according to Kitty Stryker, Good Fatties are meant to be funny. Being a Good Fatty means also being a good sport, and being able to take a slight against their own large body size. If offended by someone (non-obese) saying 'It's only a joke', a person with obesity is not playing the game – it certainly isn't a joke to them. As an anthropologist, I know that jokes can allow people to say things that can't otherwise be said in everyday polite society. Carrying excess weight is not a laughing matter, and that kind of joke is a form of bullying. While bullying is addressed with increased effect at least within institutions, in the non-institutional world, jokes against body fatness remain common. How low is that, when someone's identity is linked so tightly to their body that they are expected to take jokes at the expense of their own excess weight? As Stryker says, 'My body is not a punchline.'

Being a female Good Fatty often means living a life to please others, striving to gain approval and love by being the kind of Good Fatty at the right time. This is exhausting. Kitty Stryker has given up on being a Good Fatty, now treating eating in public as a revolutionary act. She struggles with the ways of the judgemental world she lives in. Imagine how it is for all those people who do not have her strength of character. In relation to obesity, moralizing thoughts, either external or internalized from the judgemental world, do not lead to virtuous acts.

Body Stigma Is Used to Reinforce Social Difference

Public signals of approval or disapproval are effective in establishing and maintaining common knowledge of a moral norm, and obesity stigma is a way of establishing and maintaining a moral norm around body size. If a person with obesity is stigmatized in the clinical setting, then obesity is no longer just about health, but about maintaining a moral norm, for which the BMI (for example) can be used as an instrument of moralization. Doing it publicly – shaming and blaming the person with obesity – ensures that everyone knows what the moral norm around body size is, and that everyone else knows that everyone knows what the moral norm around body size is. The BMI becomes something that helps keep the world normal for people of normal weight, and people with obesity become transgressors of the norm. If people with obesity stop listening to these moralizing discourses, they become dangerous by threatening the norm. As the numbers of people carrying excess weight grow, so the norm is progressively challenged. Maybe that's why there is such a fierce backlash against obesity in the Western world.

The inferior status attached to fat bodies in Western societies has a history going back around 300 years. During the sixteenth and seventeenth centuries, painters like Peter Paul Rubens and Jacob Jordaens (among many others) celebrated the fat European body. This was a time when the European social imaginary placed female body fatness on a pedestal. Aesthetic preferences shifted, though, with early modernity and the colonization of the world by European nations. By the eighteenth century, excessive body fatness was seen by many Europeans as being associated with a lack of intelligence, with excessive food consumption seen as an obstacle to higher thought. Post-Reformation, self-regulation became key to cultivating morality, in which gluttony was a sin. In the late eighteenth and nineteenth centuries, body fat became a resource for racial categorization, with the writings of early race scientists, such as George Cuvier, Julien-Joseph Virey, and Georges-Louis Leclerc, Comte de Buffon (known widely now as Buffon), drawing direct ties between gluttony, stupidity, and the characteristics of Africans, whose idleness was attributed to the warm climate they lived in. Such thinking was also a part of the colonial discourse about India. A thin physique became a signal of the moral and intellectual superiority of Europeans, supported by the writings of anthropologists and naturalists seeking to codify and biologize a racial hierarchy. Scientific 'race-makers' went one step further by fusing this 'ascetic aesthetic' with the moral imperative of temperance.

Discriminating against large bodies allows the 'othering' of people with obesity, negating their humanity, making them seem less worthy of dignity and respect. By othering, prejudices against people with obesity are reinforced. At a larger scale, it contributes to the potential dehumanization of people with obesity as a whole. Obesity stigma and othering is used to develop and maintain social hierarchies. There are various ways in which this happens, and I will describe three of them, starting with a common visual trope in obesity studies, the graphic representation of obesity with the 'fat (d)evolution' image.

You know it, I am sure – the fat (d)evolution image of several evolving hominin forms, from ape to *Homo erectus*, to *Homo sapiens* as hunter-gatherer, then as agriculturalist, then as slumped over a screen and extremely obese. There are several book covers that feature an image like this. According to Francis Ray White of Westminster University, this type of image parodies the iconography of the 'March of Progress', illustrating the evolution of humankind from ape to human, a book cover illustration drawn by Rudolf Zallinger and published in 1965. The fat (d)evolution image features an additional fat figure (and in some cases a final stage represented by a pig), visualising obesity as a 'kind of' devolution. Taken at face value, such images offer a shorthand for narratives of evolution, and human mismatch in relation to present-day environments that can predispose to obesity. While the intent of such images is often comedic, this parody is dangerous, since according to White, this construction of fatness is underpinned by discourses of gender, race, and class distinctions. The rhetorical success of this type of image relies on the othering of fat bodies, contributing to the dehumanization of people with excess body fatness.

A second way in which obesity stigma and othering is used to develop and maintain social hierarchy is in relation to the history of anti-Black discourses. Sabrina Strings, of the University of California, Irvine, has traced the roots of fat phobia to anti-Blackness movements in the US from the time of slavery. According to Strings, the category of 'Whiteness' was formed in opposition to the category of 'Blackness' in the course of racial formation in the US, in which Whiteness was consolidated as dominant. This not only involved the demonization of Black skin, but also identified body fat with Black femininity, being seen by White people as being both excessive and inferior.

According to Strings, as the nineteenth century gave rise to the American empire, the ideal of American beauty was created to sustain American White supremacy over immigrants and enslaved Africans. So in the American context grew thinness as an index of both racial and class distinction. More broadly, by the end of the nineteenth century, the culturally, scientifically, and religiously embedded view of excess body fatness as a sign of racial otherness, intellectual inferiority, and moral debasement set the conditions for the negative moral discourses surrounding excessive body fatness which persist to the present day.

A third way in which body fatness discourses shape and maintain social hierarchies is through the reinforcement of social class norms, especially among European populations, when social and cultural tensions of social class intersect with obesity discourses and their accompanying imperatives related to bodily discipline, physical activity, and diet. This does not extend beyond White populations, however. In Jamaica, for example, there is no singular body-size-related aesthetic, but obesity stigma exists, and experience of stigma is influenced by socioeconomic status and socioeconomic aspiration. What seems to be more widespread is the extent to which obesity hinders social mobility and is associated with downward mobility for some – in Jamaica, Sweden, and the UK, for starters.

What Can We Do?

Stigma is always rife when people want to create and maintain differences between them and others, when those differences work for them. It is worth considering who is doing the stigmatizing, and what benefits they think they gain by doing so. Inequality is a drag on many economies of wealthy nations, and it would seem sensible to reduce it. This is easier said than done, given that free-market economics relies on gradients of inequality to function. It's probably too much to expect business to set a moral lead here, but what about religion? It depends on the faith that guides you. The Q'uran steers towards moderation with 'Eat and drink, but do not be excessive' and 'He likes not those who commit excess.' The Old Testament of the Bible is morally judgemental where it warns against excess, with 'Put a knife to your throat if you are given to gluttony', and where it is also written that God withdraws his blessing from a man whose 'face is covered with fat and his waist bulges with flesh'.

Decolonization of body fatness discourses is important, in the broader global decolonization of institutions. Values linked to diverse ancestry and body fatness have racialized histories, and excess body fatness and obesity should also be part of the decolonization discourse. This is underway in studies of indigenous diet and chronic disease, mostly in relation to 'rediscovering' healthy traditional food ways. Obesity science might strive to be more in line with changing societal values, especially in promoting social justice and human rights for people of excess weight. In 2012, Joe Millward, of the

University of Surrey, titled a debate about obesity at the UK Nutrition Society 'Energy balance and obesity: a UK perspective on the gluttony *v.* sloth debate.' I find it shocking, because naming the debate in this way institutionally legitimizes the blaming and shaming of people with obesity. An individual scientist might miss this if their nose has been too close to the laboratory bench to notice a shift in societal norms, but an august institution of science should be raising awareness of the need to destigmatize and decolonize scientific practice, and of the societal damage that careless labelling can do.

The Joint International Consensus Statement for Ending Stigma of Obesity of 2020 goes some way towards doing something about obesity stigma. Led by Francesco Rubino, of King's College London, this consensus statement, and associated pledge, were agreed at a joint conference of ten Euro-American obesity based and obesity related professional organizations, including the World Obesity Federation, the Obesity Society, the European Association for the Study of Obesity, the American Association for Metabolic and Bariatric Surgery, and the International Federation for the Surgery of Obesity and Metabolic Disorders. Consensus was reached on the position that weight stigma damages health, undermines human and social rights, and is unacceptable in modern societies; and that academic institutions, professional organizations, media, public-health authorities, and governments should encourage education about weight stigma to facilitate a new public narrative about obesity, coherent with modern scientific knowledge. The statement condemns the use of stigmatizing language, images, attitudes, policies, and weight-based discrimination wherever they occur. Their pledges are given in Table 6.1. While these might help to reduce obesity stigma in professional domains if rigorously enforced, removing body-weight-based stigma in everyday life is something else. Institutional support for dealing with stigmatization of people with excess weight in everyday life is needed. Perhaps something along the lines of the UK's Tackling Racism and Racial Inequality in Sport (TRARIIS) Review of 2020. This was undertaken by the CEOs of the four governmental sports organizations and one leading arms-length body of government, with practical policies and procedures in place which are under regular review.

Existing research overwhelmingly demonstrates that obesity stigma is an ineffective way to reduce obesity and that it promotes quite the opposite – weight

Pledge 1	To treat individuals with overweight and obesity with dignity and respect.
Pledge 2	To refrain from using stereotypical language, images, and narratives that unfairly and inaccurately depict individuals with overweight and obesity as lazy, gluttonous, and lacking will power or self-discipline.
Pledge 3	To encourage and support educational initiatives aimed at eradicating weight bias through dissemination of current knowledge of obesity and body-weight regulation.
Pledge 4	To encourage and support initiatives aimed at preventing weight discrimination in the workplace, education, and healthcare settings.

From Rubino et al. (2020)

Table 6.1   Four pledges of the International Consensus Statement to eliminate weight bias and stigma of obesity (from Rubino et al. 2020)

gain. Oli Williams and Ellie Annandale, of Leicester University, have observed the perpetual uncertainty and morality that characterizes the practice of weight management. They examined the internalization of negative weight stereotypes and subsequent self-disparagement that comes from being a victim of obesity stigma, with detrimental impacts on mental and physical health. You can't change the world tomorrow, but being kinder to everyone, including people carrying excess body fatness can help. It might be a 'one brick at a time' approach, but if medical institutions are prepared to change, then individuals should do so too. If you carry excess body fat, be kind to yourself. If you know someone of excess weight, hear their story and understand their path.

7 You Eat Too Much

Space Left for Pudding

When I put on weight over Christmas, I tell myself I will burn it off in the summer, when I get out more. When summer comes around, I can't resist a barbecue and a nice glass of red wine. When I put on weight across the summer, I tell myself I will take it off come September, when I get back to serious business again. The thing is, there is never a time in the future when I can take weight off by simply watching what I eat over a short period of time, so I just have to watch myself all the time. How can I not eat too much, when there is so much good and tasty food around, and when I love my food, as I always have? This chapter considers the misunderstanding that everyone can regulate their appetite and eat only what their share is, for a stable body weight and stable energy balance. It just doesn't work like that. Some people can very easily overeat without noticeable effect, while many of us cannot and dare not, without putting on weight. All of us are given the cultural excuse to overeat on festive occasions such as Christmas and at summer picnics and barbecues, eating more than enough and fooling ourselves that we still have space left in our stomachs for pudding. Genetics and epigenetics (Chapter 2) are important predisposing factors to appetites big and small, as is the ready availability of cheap ultra-processed foods (UPFs) which goad you to eat plenty of tasty but empty calories (Chapter 4). These factors play on our physiology and metabolism in interconnected ways that stimulate overeating, often quite situationally. In this chapter, I examine the evolutionarily based ability of most people to easily overeat and be attracted to energy-dense foods, noting that not all calories are equal in human metabolism (Chapter 3). Fats may contain more calories, but eating refined carbohydrates (including sugar) more usually results in fat deposition in places that may do harm (Chapter 1). Food is plentiful in most parts of the world, notwithstanding hunger in some parts. UPFs are ubiquitous, and I go on to consider why we as humans are drawn to them, finishing with some thoughts about how we might keep our appetites under control, despite all the factors that operate against it.

A Hominin in the Modern World

I like a nice barbecue, with my plate spilling over with foods high in fat and protein, charred and salty, mouth-drippingly tasty, at least to my senses. These days I don't light the barbecue for a family meal because I see it as a licence for everyone to let go of their food inhibitions and eat plentifully, often beyond full, feasting not eating. Thinking about it, if I were a hominin around a million years ago, I would welcome it with open arms. Charring flesh on an open fire – 'What's not to like?' My ancestral hominin me would eat until full, beyond being replete, because who knows what I might find to eat tomorrow? Eating at a barbecue now brings back the deeply engrained early hunter-gatherer response to food plenty – eating like there is no tomorrow, because tomorrow, who knows? There may be no food. These days, we may wear business suits and pantyhose and fine shoes, but underneath all of this finery is a deeply insecure hominin that responds to all kinds of life stresses by reaching for a tasty snack and maybe more. Extra calories can both fill the adipose tissue in readiness for future food insecurity and placate the psychological insecurity that is generated by all kinds of stresses that bombard us in everyday life. The trouble is that the food system as it is configured right now, from production to processing and preparation to distribution and retail, is mostly geared toward supplying cheap calories. Producing enough calories to feed the world's growing population was a major issue maybe 70 years ago or so, but globally, the world food system has largely risen to resolve this challenge since then. Food prices rose sharply across the board at the start of the Russia–Ukraine war, but now well over a year into the conflict they have pulled back considerably, and foods rich in refined carbohydrates remain cheap when compared with most other foods on the market. According to the Food and Agriculture Organization of the United Nations, just prior to the COVID-19 pandemic and the Russia–Ukraine war, people across the world had on average 36% more calories available to them than in 1961, 31% more calories from wheat, and a staggering 85% more fat.

Admittedly, the 1960s were a time when undernutrition and starvation were much more pressing problems than overnutrition (more is said about this in relation to nutrition transition in Chapter 4). Now, obesity has become a nutritional issue of major proportion in both the Global North and the Global South, something that was not envisaged back then. So what is our inner hominin to do, in a world of multiple stresses, where food shortage is no longer a major problem, and where in most parts of the world the easiest way of reducing stress is to comfort-eat the tasty foods that so easily translate into inches on the hips, thighs, or belly? A starting point might be to look at what lies upstream, at those things that cause us to overeat. The immediate gratifications of overeating are often inconsistent with the longer-term gratifications of health and achieving normative bodily ideals (mostly muscular thin ones, these days).

We can never leave our evolutionary selves behind, however sophisticated we might think we are. We have evolved foraging strategies that are ecologically based, involving embedded approaches to obtaining food and to eating that involve perceptions of risks and benefits. Our eating behaviours are evolutionarily rational, even if they are often out of kilter with traditional and contemporary cultures surrounding food, its preparation, and its consumption. Our understandings of risk attached to eating are also often out of kilter with changing food consumption patterns in the world now, but we do not easily intuit this, especially when the health risks, such as cardiovascular disease and type 2 diabetes, are many years downstream. Without feeding there is no survival, and we have evolved neural and hormonal mechanisms in the neocortex of the brain to survive through creating and maintaining associative pleasures in food. As humans we express these mechanisms (through genetics, epigenetics, and behaviour) to a much higher degree than any other species. In the evolutionary past this was good, because it ensured species survival through lean times as well as times of plenty. Finding pleasure in food and satisfaction in eating is thus a fundamental evolutionary adaptation that has done us well in the past, but which is now challenged with rising obesity.

Palatability, satiation (physiological cues to terminate eating), and satiety (the feeling of fullness that often develops after eating) gained from foods are inversely related to their energy density. The doughnut in Chapter 4 is very dense in energy, and I can easily eat it so quickly that I still feel hungry after, with enthusiasm for another doughnut (and maybe another after that). I can overeat on doughnuts without realising it. Give me a bowl of porridge, though, and I won't eat it nearly as quickly. It will satisfy my appetite as I eat, and I won't be tempted by another bowlful. Food intake is driven by cognitive factors as well as by hunger and the desire for calories. There are feed-forward mechanisms between the brain and gut that anticipate the nutritional needs of the body by responding to food cues in the environment, such as the perceived qualities of potential foods (including their smell, and associations with pleasure, displeasure, or disgust), our mental expectations from them, and their sensory properties while being eaten. The regulation of appetite intersects with physiological systems that regulate pleasure and reward. For example, the appetite-regulating hormone leptin is known to inhibit sweet-sensitive taste cells in the tongue. As you eat and as your hunger is assuaged, your leptin levels rise and your perception of the sweetness of food declines. This contributes to the decline in eating across the course of an eating event (like a meal) because the food being eaten is sensed in the brain as being less palatable, even though its composition hasn't changed.

We have a mismatch between our fundamental biology, which has evolved to want to eat and find satisfaction in calories, and food production systems that provide calories easily and cheaply. So how does all this internal calorie satisfaction work deep down in the body, and does it matter where your calories come from?

Not All Calories Are Equal

Wilbur Atwater was the first person to talk about the nutritional equivalence of calories. That is, that a gram of carbohydrate contains 4 calories of dietary energy to be used in metabolism, as does a gram of protein, whereas a gram of fat contains 9 calories. On this basis, you might want to avoid fat if you want to avoid eating too many calories, given the implicit equivalence of macronutrient calories implied by the Atwater Factors of 4, 4, and 9 calories of food

energy per gram of carbohydrate, protein, and fat, respectively. This equivalence has worked well in helping scientists and planners determine national
food requirements and in guiding national food requirements, but it doesn't
work so well at the level of the individual. I have just moved office, and this has
involved shifting over 2,000 books, deciding which remain important to me,
which are to stay in the Department, which to bring home to my studio at
home, which to donate to the Oxfam bookshop in central Oxford. One of the
books I have managed to avoid for over 30 years while it has been on my
bookshelf is a report of the Select Committee on Nutrition and Human Needs
of the United States (US) Senate, on Dietary Goals. I flicked through it, out of
curiosity more than anything, and found something interesting. On obesity, it
states that in relation to weight control, fat is recognized as the most concentrated source of food energy, suggesting that to avoid weight gain, citizens of
the US should eat less fat. That was in 1977. That advice, to eat less fat, has not
helped in achieving weight loss among the US population across the decades
since it was published. Patricia Nguyen of Stanford University, and her colleagues, compared fat-free, low-fat, and regular versions of the same processed foods using data collected from the United States Department of
Agriculture National Nutrient Database, and found that both low-fat and fat-
free versions are loaded with much more sugar than the regular versions of
those foods. Displacing dietary fat with carbohydrate (rather than just removing fat) in foods and encouraging people to eat those foods might have had the
opposite effect to that intended, which was to help people put on more weight,
rather than take it off. Isn't fact sometimes stranger than fiction? In hindsight,
there is a good explanation, so let me explain.

Not all people are born equal, and not all calories are equal. Believing that
they are led to a crazy outcome, especially in the US where for generations
people have been urged to reduce their intake of fat so as to reduce their total
intake of calories. In 2018, David Ludwig and Cara Ebbeling, of the Harvard
Medical School, published a critique of conventional decades-long
approaches to obesity treatments which assume that all calories are metabolically alike, and that to lose weight people should eat fewer calories and
be more physically active. Trying to lose weight by restricting calories
increases hunger and reduces energy expenditure, both of which run coun-
ter to weight loss, and it did not surprise Ludwig and Ebbeling that following

the energy-balance dictum fails the individual in the long run, even if it might succeed in promoting weight loss in the short term. Even when people manage to lose weight by counting calories in and calories out, most eventually put it back on again.

Human energy-balance regulation is more tolerant of positive than negative energy balance, and it is a lot easier to gain weight than to lose it. Energy balance might be homeostatically regulated, but when it fluctuates (which in most people it does, frequently if irregularly), there is progressive deposition of body fat through a steady retention of energy. Energy expenditure is a major determinant of appetite and the human physiological drive to eat. Ludwig and colleagues have proposed an alternative way of looking at the physiology of calories coming into the body. This is the carbohydrate–insulin model, in which overeating is not seen as driving body fat increase over the long term, but rather, the process of storing excess body fat is seen to drive overeating. High intakes of processed carbohydrates, like sugar and things made with refined wheat flour, elicit a range of hormonal responses that promote storage of energy in adipose tissue and leave fewer calories for muscular work and metabolic activity across other tissues of the body, making for a sense of hunger while at the same time depositing body fat. Calorie-bearing carbohydrates are seen as tricking the body into feeling hungry while at the same time reducing energy expended in metabolic rate as the body senses carbohydrate-induced starvation and attempts to conserve energy. This effect need only be very small indeed, less than 20 calories per day, for slow but progressive weight gain.

There are other ways in which not all calories are equal, especially when it comes to appetite and satiety. James Stubbs, of the University of Leeds, has spent much of his life showing how protein, carbohydrate, and fat intakes have a hierarchy of effect on satiety, with the former being the most filling, and the latter the least filling but also the most energy-dense of the macronutrients. By increasing the energy density of food with fat, people can easily consume calories without satisfying their appetite as easily as if they were eating protein-rich foods, and therefore run the risk of overeating relative to physiological energy requirements and gaining weight.

Food liking and wanting, and learning about how different foods make you feel are central to personal eating patterns, as are the hedonic and physiological mechanisms that make different types of foods more, or less, palatable. There are times when it is all too easy to overeat. Leaving aside stress and comfort eating (Chapter 6), people often eat more in social contexts and at events when it is deemed socially OK to overeat, like during festivals such as Christmas. External cues, like branding, advertising, and ways in which food offerings are presented for purchase and consumption, also promote overeating through influences on food choice and patterns of eating. The macronutrient composition of food also influences its liking and intake. While fat on its own is not pleasant to eat, it is a taste stimulus that doesn't vary according to emotion, unlike sweetness. We like the taste of fat much more when it is in complex food combinations, especially when there is sugar there, even in small amounts. When you put fat and sugar together, the combination of sweetness and high fat encourages overeating to a much greater extent than any other macronutrient combination. The evolutionarily based human preference for energy-dense, palatable foods consisting of a mix of macronutrients is easily exploited by food manufacturers and retailers.

Food Availability in the Modern World

A hominin a million years ago would not immediately be able to thrive off supermarket foods, simply because the packaging and labelling would not offer honest signals of the energy density of those foods. However, if they experimented with them – these packaged, branded foods – they would quickly thrive once they worked out what was tasty to eat and what was not. Then they would likely over-consume, and put on weight as the anticipated seasonal shortfall of food usual in hominin life would not happen. Place yourselves in the shoes of that early hominin in the supermarket. You are able to adapt to extremes of diet, to live in a climate of food security risk, but your hominin food-life is so comfortable that it will kill you slowly. That's where most people in the Global North are now – being slowly killed by comfort.

Humans evolved in tropical Africa, where seasonality mostly consists of wet and dry seasons. As hominins moved to the top of the food chain, being able to consume nature at all levels, from plants (including roots, shoots, and fruits) to insects and animals small and large, seasonal environments created huge amounts of diversity in both types of potential foods available at any time, and of overall availability of food. As modern humans migrated out of Africa around 70,000 years ago, so they were exposed to different ecologies and changing patterns of seasonality, to which they mostly adapted, changing their foraging and eating patterns according to environmental limitations. Thus, humans became able to consume the widest diversity of plant and animal foods of all mammals, while still sharing the tendency to overeat in response to food portion size, palatability, and energy density with other mammals, an evolutionary trait that is favoured in seasonal environments where scarcity is common (Chapter 2). Most mammals are able to overeat to high levels of body fatness, indicating that at least some of the genetic basis for human obesity lies in evolutionary time that is deeper than that of the hominin–chimpanzee divergence of over 7 million years ago. We also share the biological drives of feeding, hunger, and the dietary regulation of macronutrient intake with other animals beyond the primates, as well as the social facilitation of food intake, where social interaction increases the amounts of food eaten at an eating event, when food is plentiful. What limits food intake for humans are individual, social, and cultural constraints.

While seasonality remains an environmental pressure for many human popu-lations currently living in traditional ways involving rural subsistence, this has largely disappeared for modern humans, food availability in a global food system offering a consistent supply of food types regardless of the time of year. Francis Fukuyama, then at the Rand Corporation, Santa Monica, California, famously wrote of the end of history, of a world where liberal democracy would prevail everywhere, and where politics as we know it would be reduced to mere management. In 1992, the time of publication of Fukuyama's book, global food security was also moving toward its own type of 'end of history', in which undernutrition would be conquered, and nutrition transition (Chapter 4) would move people toward nutritional enlightenment when all would eat healthily, and diseases both infectious and chronic would become a thing of the past. It didn't work out that way, neither for Fukuyama's prediction, nor for food security and extremes of nutrition, both under- and over-, largely because human societies do not remain stable, nor do human appetites. Lack of food seasonality in type and quantity of food is an important contributor to obesity (inasmuch as there is no shortage of food at any given time of year), alongside the human appetite for dietary diversity, sweetness, fat, protein, and overall palatability.

Food availability is often estimated by what is sold, but knowing what is eaten where, and understanding how food is chosen and how its materiality is turned into bodily metabolism, are also important for understanding how obesity is produced, as are the dynamics of eating. For example, some people eat in isolation, some eat socially, and both can be good or bad in measure. Moreover, most people eat at home most of the time, and while most of what is bought in a store is taken home and eaten there, there is less knowledge of who eats what within a home, although consumption of UPFs is known to be bad for health regardless of how what is bought is distributed.

Why Do We Like Ultra-Processed Foods?

Why we like UPFs is down to evolutionarily based drives and the food cues we respond to, most of which we learn from a very young age. At any given moment our responses to food cues are highly stable, but are heavily determined by social contexts of eating, as well as expectations from the foods we plan to eat. In the absence of food limitation in either volume, weight, or energy, the most powerful behavioural influences on the amounts of what we eat are: other individuals at a meal; watching something on a screen; the size of food packages; portion size; palatability; energy density; and the consumption of caloric beverages with a meal. Food novelty plays its part too. Many industrial food products are designed to appeal to the palate as well as being energy-dense, and the range of tasty energy-dense UPFs marketed in wealthy countries has grown enormously across in the past 40 years or so. The constant development of new foods designed to appeal to the senses has contributed to the separation of sensory from nutritional attributes of foods in ways that inhibit learning what is good to eat by associative conditioning through palatability, appetite, and satiety. We like UPFs because they are tasty and they make us feel good. Deep-down, our brain is convinced we are eating good food, but we are being tricked because we no longer know how to work out what good nutritious food is, from its sensory properties alone.

In the US, portion sizes of prepackaged and restaurant-prepared foods increased hugely in the late twentieth century. In many wealthy countries, snacking between meals has increased and meals have become increasingly de-structured across the same period. Snack foods are often densely caloric, prepared, processed, and packaged, and people often snack without feeling physically hungry, especially when distracted by an external stimulus, like using a screen. The digital world also offers extensive exposure to commercial marketing of energy-dense foods.

UPFs have characteristics that favour the development of obesity, including being of high energy density, with high fat and fructose content. Time constraints on home cooking in wealthy countries are also part of this, with the emergence and rise in demand for prepackaged convenience foods with short preparation times, with more food being consumed away from the home. Other time-saving devices, such as drive-through, 24-hour, take-away, and home-delivery food services have helped make food ubiquitous in everyday life in wealthy countries and helped the spread of UPFs. But UPFs are also to be found across the Global South, as was very evident in the Cook Islands when I worked there in 1995, and emergent in rural Papua New Guinea in the 1980s. In poorer countries, many UPFs are marketed to appeal to people's aspirations to modernity. Which leaves us where we are now – with UPFs penetrating all aspects of the retail-end of the food system almost everywhere.

Palatability, Appetite, and Self-Control

As energy-dense and (in combination) palatable macronutrients, fat and sugar have become increasingly available in recent decades as well as being implicated in the production of obesity. The desire to eat sugar is reinforced behaviourally and physiologically, inducing pleasure through the neuronal release of opioids. 'Aren't opioids addictive?' I can hear you say. Well, yes, but there are different levels of addiction, and firm evidence is needed before we can say that sugar is addictive.

James DiNicolantonio, of Saint Luke's Mid-America Heart Institute, Kansas City, has sifted the evidence for sugar addiction, concluding from animal studies that the regular consumption of added sugars gives a number of drug-like effects, including bingeing; craving; tolerance; and withdrawal. There are substantial parallels and overlaps in brain neurochemistry and behaviour of individuals (animal and human) using drugs of abuse, and of those eating sugar. Sugar addiction, according to DiNicolantonio, is real because the endogenous opioids released in the brain after eating sugar are similar to those released after drug use.

It's not all down to addictiveness, though. There is a social element to eating, with social regulation being less powerful in individualist societies than in communitarian ones, like Japan, for example. In the absence of socially calibrating checks and balances, cheap, palatable, energy-dense food can easily be overconsumed regardless of social context – for stress alleviation or for pleasure, or both combined. Feelings of uncertainty and anxiety encourage overeating, and people put on weight in response to stress, whether due to subordinate status, inequality, work insecurity, or financial insecurity. Anxiety rates remain high in many wealthy countries and especially so in the US, where palatable UPFs form a legal means of self-medication. The US has seen increased energy intakes from snacking, while energy intakes from meals have remained constant across recent decades. In countries that place great emphasis on maintaining a strong meal structure – Japan again – there is less snacking, which limits energy intake both socially and culturally. In an age when another way of dealing with anxiety through distraction – smoking – is strongly frowned upon and disincentivized through taxation, and in the absence of other forms of emotional support, consumption of cheap UPFs can provide comfort by reducing negative emotions such as anger, boredom, and depression. Eating high-fat diets also reduces sensitivity to stress as well as reducing stress itself, although there are withdrawal symptoms associated with reducing fat intake, which can elevate stress again and increase the desire to eat a high-fat diet.

In societies promoting individualist values, the regulation of obesity is often synonymous with individual self-control, and models for obesity regulation overwhelmingly focus on responsibility and self-management: for eating healthily; maintaining a healthy body weight; and undertaking adequate physical activity. 'Responsibilized' consumer citizenship places the task of resisting palatable, highly energy-dense foods upon the individual (Chapter 5), but according to Elinor Ochs and Carolina Izquierdo, of the University of California, Los Angeles, wealthier people are more able to self-regulate than poorer ones, and are less likely to engage the powerful behavioural urges to eat in response to food cues. These differences are likely to be due to differences in social and economic capital (Chapter 5) – the more agency you have in life, the more likely you are to be able to self-regulate.

Let's turn now to appetite and its regulation. This hasn't had the time, in an evolutionary sense, to adapt to the food environment created by corporate interests, rich in cheap UPFs which signal attractiveness through branding and labelling. Two theories have been proposed to explain between-individual differences in food consumption behaviours and the tendency to overeat. The first, that of externality, views people with obesity to be more reactive to external cues (such as the time of day, presence of food, and situational effects) and less sensitive to internal physiological hunger and satiety signals than are non-obese people. The second theory, of psychosomatic feeding, focuses on the role of emotion in guiding eating patterns. The usual response to arousal (such as fear, anxiety, or anger) is loss of appetite, but some people respond by overeating.

Behaviours associated with obesity – eating more dietary energy than is expended, over prolonged periods, eating refined carbohydrates which deposit fat abdominal more readily and elicit hunger easily – have a number of potential rewards, including pleasure, distraction, and relief from stress and anxiety. Most societies are, to varying degree, embedded in cultures of consumption now, especially in the Global North where many aspects of personal identity are forged through what people buy and have. Many of the factors that are seen as having contributed to obesity across recent decades involve consumption, not only of highly energy-dense food and drink, but of other goods and services, including motor cars, personal computers, and electronic devices, all of which facilitate increased convenience and promote further increased consumption.

Checks and balances to overeating include the many social conventions surrounding food and its consumption in all societies. These are quite easily overridden, however, especially in individualist societies like the UK and the US. Eating while listening to the radio or watching media, or eating in the presence of friends and family, increases the amount consumed. Both sets of circumstances allow diversion of attention from food consumption, resulting in reduced self-monitoring of intake, allowing food consumption beyond immediate needs. Engaging in other tasks, such as working and playing at the computer, also reduces self-monitoring of food intake. Online activity has been shown to shape eating behaviours, bodily dissatisfaction, and physical activity patterns, in ways that can damage health. Obesity travels through social networks, and three interrelated processes are viewed to drive this process. These are: social contagion (whereby the network in which a person is embedded influences their weight or weight-influencing behaviours); social capital (whereby a sense of belonging and of having social support influences a person's weight or weight-influencing behaviours); and social selection (whereby a person's network develops according to their weight – if they put on weight, they will assort with people who also put on weight). These factors almost certainly change in importance across the course of someone's life, and being in a social network that promotes or is permissive of excess body weight is not destiny. However, new digital media are evolving fast, television is almost a thing of the past, and new platforms and digital devices are proliferating, changing these networked relationships. Diverse mobile technologies (since 2004) and the Internet of Things (since 2014) are disrupting and changing most aspects of society, including how food is consumed. Individualism, modern life, engagement with the digital world, and the proliferation of cheap UPFs make disordered, disregulated, and distracted eating easy to practise. So, what can we do?

What Can We Do?

The global food system is the most significant upstream contributor to human nutrition in most societies, and food has never been as cheap or as plentiful as in the past few decades. Among the cheapest foods are those based on agricultural commodities, especially cereals, sugars, and edible oils, which are easy to overconsume relative to energetic need, and which are produced in great quantity by the global food system. The commercial processed food system has many facets and is illustrated in the broadest way in relation to the production of obesity in Figure 7.1. Its multiple components are mostly cogs in the market economy mechanism, through the operation of individual but often interdependent companies and corporations. Truth be told, most of the food system lies beyond government control, and perhaps that is why

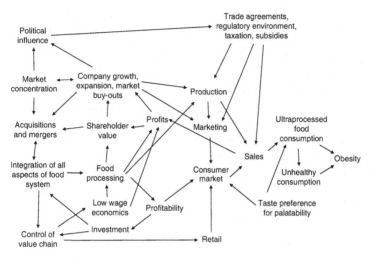

Figure 7.1   The commercial processed food system and obesity.

governments generally do not intervene in food systems to any great extent anymore. At the political level, the individual is largely unprotected from corporate UPFs.

If we can't control big food, can we medicate against obesity? Wouldn't it be nice if you could just pop a pill every day and this would reduce your appetite? No longer would you have to fight the cravings for sugar and other foods that are easily overeaten and can lead to weight gain. The search for anti-obesity medication has a long history, mostly focused on increasing energy expenditure, and overwhelmingly failing in its quest. More recent developments in drug therapy of obesity have focused on appetite regulation. Semaglutide is an analogue of the hormone GLP-1 which reduces energy intake, reduces hunger, and increases feelings of satiety. Sounds perfect – does it work? It seems to, but it's not a pill, but a weekly subcutaneous injection. At the time of writing, it has been approved for use in Canada, Europe, the UK, and the US to complement a reduced calorie diet and increased physical activity for people classified as having obesity, or being overweight with at least one chronic disease condition. But the downside is that, according to John Wilding, of the University of Liverpool, and his colleagues, within a year of stopping this medication, most people regain two-thirds of the weight lost. It is clearly not for everyone.

Governments may not want to, but we can call on them to do more in terms of regulating the food system, for example by more stringently controlling the marketing of UPFs or making them more expensive through taxation. The sugar-sweetened beverage (SSB) tax in the UK has led to some reduction in sugar consumption without reducing corporate profits, so there is hope. Such taxation, in the UK and elsewhere, also helps in nudging the companies that make such products to reformulate towards healthier ones. With respect to sugar, this usually involves replacing it with artificial sweeteners, some of which have been approved for use by the US Food and Drug Administration – saccharin, sucralose, aspartame, neotame, and cyclamate. This remains a controversial issue, however, some experts calling for more evidence of their safety for health.

Food is still most often framed by governments as being a consumerist issue, and it is far easier to focus on individual-level factors and place responsibility for obesity on this, as most policy responses have for decades. The current logic of individualism in obesity prevention and treatment in the UK, the US, and Australia is consumerist, perhaps because the global food system, among other commercially dominated systems, relies on consumption for its demand. Taxation runs the risk of simply making UPFs more expensive, which, in the absence of cheap healthy alternatives, is likely to swallow a greater proportion of the budgets of poorer people, for whom such foods make up a substantial proportion of their diets.

If governments duck the responsibility of regulating food systems, or feel unable to do so, can food corporations be persuaded to act more responsibly? Clare Herrick, of King's College London, has argued that food and drinks industries use health as a corporate social responsibility strategy to maintain brand value and consumer goodwill, in response to governmental and public calls in the US and the UK for higher levels of accountability. This has been termed 'health-washing', a corporate marketing ploy that gives a false impression of healthiness to food products (often without claims being confirmed as true), allowing them to maintain or grow sales in a market that demands more from them. The food industry often uses very specific interpretations of health in its view of corporate social responsibility. For example, industry strategies that promote narrow epidemiological understandings of obesity may divert attention away from specific foods (which they produce) to diet (which consumers construct by combining different foods produced by a wide range of companies). Focusing on diets deflects attention away from obesogenic foods that are designed, produced, marketed, and sold by food corporations, to diets, which are more a matter of individual choice. They also dilute any regulatory action a government might take in relation to such foods.

Policy that calls on people to take responsibility for their health through their eating actions is appealing – amounting to minimal political intervention – but has limited impact on obesity rates. Alternatively, the regulation of food systems by governments involves many competing interests and is politically difficult, but is more likely to be effective. There are several conflicting interests in regulating food systems. Governments seek to have healthy and economically productive citizens, whereas food corporations seek profit. And citizens often respond to policies and market forces individualistically.

As a species, we are extremely reactive to social evaluation, and use our emotions to guide us through the world, perhaps more so than rational thinking. Emotion is strongly implicated in overeating and obesity, as well as in decision-making in many other aspects of life. People rely on affective reactions, positive or negative, to speed up judgements and decision-making, and these can sometimes predispose to obesity in the longer term. For example, eating when you are happy or satisfied with life is more likely to be associated with healthy food behaviours and choices than eating when you are unhappy. Biology is unconcerned about health and well-being beyond its contribution to reproductive fitness and reduced mortality, however, and the procurement, processing, and consumption of food are all evolutionarily rational practices that influence reproductive success and survival. We can be aware of the forces stacked against us in trying to eat in a healthy way and not gain weight, and can still act with agency in our everyday food choices. Eating for pleasure – hedonic hunger – has an evolutionary basis, and this mechanism has been deliberately hijacked by the parts of the food industry whose business is to produce and retail highly palatable, energy-dense foods. Most of us have a physiology that defends our body weight and a behavioural tendency to overeat when faced with anxiety and insecurity, both of which have an evolutionary basis. You can't fault the structure of human metabolism, only the circumstances in which it is being asked to operate.

8 You Don't Get Out Enough

Walking Off the Chocolate Bar

How much exercise does it take to walk off an average single-person-sized chocolate bar? More than you might want to acknowledge, even though you probably already know that. No chocolate bar is calorie-free, and if you are an average-sized woman in the UK, eating a 100-gram chocolate bar will take around two hours of walking to burn off. In this chapter, I examine the idea that people put on excess weight because they don't get enough physical activity. Most people in Western societies don't get out enough, so why stigmatize a person with obesity for not being physically active? Sure, physical activity is great, especially for reducing stress, staying happy, and lowering blood pressure and other risk markers of chronic disease, but not especially so for burning calories and keeping body weight down. The best thing about regular exercise is that it helps you burn off and keep off the wrong kind of fat, the kind that can make you long-term ill. It also helps you eat to your energy requirement more closely than if you don't exercise. I can see that from data collected in the first UK COVID-19 lockdown by myself and my colleagues, published in an Insight Report to the UK Parliament. You probably don't want to remember it – those months when people hardly got out, felt unhappy, snacked more, and many put on weight. Although most people want to be physically active, the ability to be so is influenced by environmental factors such as the availability of pavements and sidewalks, by green and blue spaces, and by stage of life – young children want to be far more active than people in their eighties, for example.

Public health uses the rubric of physical activity as a butterfly net to attempt to capture the integration of complex behaviours associated with human move-ment and relate them to measures of health and illness. Physical activity is the most variable part of total energy expenditure (more about this in Chapter 3) and comprises the activities of daily living, which include occupational ones, active transportation, and household work, reduced by physiologists to the term 'non-exercise activity thermogenesis' (NEAT), as well as structured exer-cise, like going for a walk or a run or a swim. The term NEAT came into being in the early 2000s, when sedentary occupations in wealthier countries became more common than physically active ones.

Social, cultural, and physical contexts are key to human movement habits and patterns. Most people live in built environments, and these have a range of spatial levels, from the very local, involving the immediate interactions of individuals with the domestic and work space around them, to buildings, neighbourhoods, and districts, to metropolitan areas big and small. In wealthy countries, patterns of physical activity in built environments are changing faster than at any time prior to the 2000s, as the digital world has been increasingly recruited to aspects of human movement – social media (Chapters 4 and 6), smart devices, and the increasing urban smartness that has come with the Internet of Things. While such changes mostly enable increased physical activity, material and social structures that make life convenient and energy-efficient at the individual level continue to reduce NEAT and promote obesity. These recent social-technological changes involving the digital world are rendering much of the pre-Web 2.0 research less currently valid, but more historically important in relation to research on obesity and the life-course (Chapter 2), which relies on understanding experiences, behaviours, and actions in early life in the subsequent development of obesity. In this chapter, I examine the human need for physical activity from an evolutionary perspective, consider evidence that physical activity matters for weight loss and weight main-tenance, and discuss how urbanism now influences physical activity patterns.

Evolution, Society, and Physical Activity

For most of our evolutionary past, humans have been foragers, subsisting on plants and animals gathered and hunted in the wild (Chapter 7). This required physical work, although the amount our hominin ancestors undertook is likely to have been small when compared with early agriculturalists. According to Robert Malina and Bertis Little, of the University of Texas at Austin and Tarleton State University, the ways of life of later hominins and early humans included regular physical activity in hunting and gathering, with a mix of continuous and intermittent work ranging between light, moderately vigorous, and occasional intense activity. While scholars now reference the Venus of Willendorf (Figure 8.1) as material symbol of fertility with her very generous waist and breasts, a person with obesity was almost certainly very rare in the Palaeolithic era. She might have had monogenic obesity, Cushing's disease, hypothyroidism, or pituitary dysfunction, but was most likely a symbol of the desirability of body fatness before the origins of agriculture.

The transition to agriculture around 10,000 years ago in different parts of the world saw widespread adoption of crop planting and animal husbandry. Dietary diversity declined dramatically for most populations, leading eventually to most groups subsisting on a very small range of plant and animal species, which involved more intensive work and physical activity than previously. As human populations grew on the back of increased dietary energy capture, the need for more food led to increased workloads as periods of activity increased and periods of rest declined. Seasonality, whether of rainfall or temperature, or both, which had guided subsistence patterns for

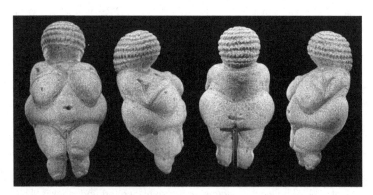

Figure 8.1   The Venus of Willendorf.

hunter-gatherers previously, now systematized work patterns for agricultural-ists according to the types of plants and animals they domesticated.

With industrialization, initially from around 270 years ago, time and physical activity of individuals came to be bought and sold to a much higher extent than in the agricultural systems that preceded it. Long hours of physical work precluded periods of rest for the emergent working classes. Those at the top of the social and economic pile engaged in physical labour to a much, much lower extent, if at all. Historical accounts of obese people in industrializing countries were usually from the wealth-ier sectors of society. Less wealthy was Daniel Lambert of Leicester, who moved to London and charged people to come and see his large body size, so unusual was it in the early 1800s.

Physical activity of pre-industrial populations was not an isolated aspect of life as it became in many industrializing, industrialized, and post-industrial econ-omies. Ever since industrialization, we have become mostly distanced from our sources of food production, selling our time, knowledge, and work, and buying our food. Foraging in the supermarket is not the same as foraging in the Kalahari Desert. Even poorer people in wealthy countries are able to forage a week's worth of calories in less than a couple of hours, something that would take Kalahari bushpeople most of the week. As a species, then, we are biological equipped for physically active lives, but are also culturally disposed to make the most of inactivity. With work mostly being mechanized and sedentary now, we can take all opportunities to be physically inactive – it is not an aberration, to want to maximize sedentariness.

Across the past 70 years or so, technologies focused on labour-saving have further reduced physical activity and energy expenditure in most settings. Occupations have become increasingly chair-bound and desk-bound, and body weights and obesity rates have increased. Across the same time frame, the privileges of being at the top of the pile, including being physically inactive and being able to eat refined foods, have trickled down to the general popula-tion in many parts of the world. Many people can enjoy being sedentary, and in wealthy countries there is little need among most people to engage in physical activity for economic purpose. As most people in wealthy countries can avail themselves of a sedentary life, physical activity – rather than inactivity – has now become a marker of status for many. Through sport, physical activity has become a way of showing prestige and distinction, because body work takes time, money, and effort.

Physical Activity and Body Weight

Does the trend toward declining levels of physical activity for the general population matter for obesity? In terms of burning calories, probably not very much. Going from being inactive to being moderately physically active means burning maybe 250 to 300 calories per day more, which, if not compensated for by increased energy intake, could lead to weight loss of over 10 kilograms across a year. What does happen is that you usually compensate increased physical activity with increased appetite, at least to some degree. If alternatively you eat less, you are likely to become lethargic and reduce energy expenditure through reduced basal metabolic rate and physical activity. An experiment carried out during the Second World War first demonstrated this. Under the direction of Ancel Keys , the Minnesota Starvation Experiment took 32 adult male conscientious objectors and semi-starved them by putting them on a diet of half of their usual daily calories for 24 weeks. They didn't lose nearly as much weight as you might think, losing on average a quarter of their body weight and not half of it as had been expected. Their basal metabolic rate dropped by around two-fifths while their energy expenditure in physical activity dropped by over a half. Keys and colleagues discovered what is now considered commonplace – that if you try to reduce weight by reducing your calorie intake, your physiology defends your body energy stores, preventing shifts in body mass.

Herman Pontzer, then of Hunter College, New York City, and his colleagues, have shown recently that humans adapt to changing diet and physical activity by adjusting behaviour and metabolism, often in quite subtle ways. In an international comparison of total energy expenditure (TEE) and physical activity, they found that TEE correlated with physical activity, but especially strongly among the least active participants. This indicates that even small changes in physical activity behaviour among the most inactive people have big implications for their TEE. Pontzer and colleagues developed what they called a constrained model of TEE, in which energy allocation among physiological tasks responds dynamically to long-term shifts in physical activity, adapting to maintain TEE within a relatively narrow range. Similarly, Rodrigo Fernandez-Verdejo of the Pontificia Universidad Católica de Chile, and his colleague Monica Suarez-Reyes of the Universidad de Santiago de Chile, observed that people who move their bodies more in walking and running adjust their TEE downwards by moving their arms less. James Levine at the Mayo Clinic and Foundation in Rochester, New York, found that fidgeting while sitting down increases energy expenditure by half again above that while just lying down, and by twice as much when standing. There is a lot of variation in this – some people are almost born to fidget if they can't move around, while others are not – but in respect of burning calories in the context of plenty, fidgeting is a good thing. Think back to your childhood days at school, where being chained to the desk was a form of slavery, where the best you could do was to tap your heels, or rock back and forth on the chair or shake a leg, sometimes two, repeatedly up and down. Your body knew it needed more activity than it was getting, and it found covert ways of getting some. Now, at my standing desk at the University of Oxford, I can stand and fidget all I like, and am doing so while writing this book. We have not evolved to sit on chairs, and that may be one reason why we don't get enough physical activity, even while we might fidget to compensate for it. Once a privilege of wealthy classes, chairs are part of everyday life for most people. Prolonged sitting down, for hours at a time, contributes to metabolic diseases such as type 2 diabetes and cardiovascular disease, even if evidence for its association with obesity is mixed. How long will it be before chairs get to carry a metabolic health warning?

While working hard physically can raise your appetite and make you want to eat more, lower levels of physical activity can fine-tune your appetite, so that what you eat is more in line with your energy expenditure. Physical activity promotes health more than it does a healthy weight, although it does help, if you are on a weight-loss diet, to exercise as well as eat fewer calories. But once you have lost weight, there isn't much strong evidence for the value of exercise in maintaining your new lower weight, even though many weight-loss gurus and organizations assert that it is more important for maintenance than for initial weight loss.

The prime site of fat deposition if consuming more calories than are being spent when physically inactive is around the gut. Gut fat – visceral fat – is more metabolically active than subcutaneous fat (Chapter 3), contributing to inflammation, or meta-inflammation, often years before full-blown chronic disease knocks at the door. Obesity is associated with chronic disease mostly because of its pro-inflammatory effects on the endocrine and immune systems. Weight loss and regular exercise protect against these effects. Being fit and having a healthy active heart allows people to perform high-intensity exercise for longer, and this can counteract the negative health consequences of excess body fatness. Vigorous aerobic exercise can lead to lower total body fat and visceral fat, and less internal fat within the abdomen, as Francisco Ortega of the University of Grenada, Spain, and his colleagues, have found.

The Built Environment

By the turn of the twenty-first century, cities, towns, rural hinterlands, and untamed wilderness areas of the world had become integrally bound to urban places through proximity and linkage. Urbanism is integral to how most people live now. Urbanization has been linked to obesity through the creation of obesogenic environments – reduced physical activity, increased availability of fast foods, greater convenience, and so on. This may well be in relation to particular urban (and suburban) forms that favour the motor car and convenience. These grew in the 1950s to the 1980s in most wealthy countries, extending into rural areas since then, as they have grown in population. The international NCD Risk Factor Collaboration has since shown that the majority of the global rise in mean BMI since the 1980s has been rural areas across the world, overwhelmingly so in poorer countries. In the US, obesity is now higher in rural than in urban areas, being associated more closely with sociodemographic factors than with urbanism. Since the early 2000s, poverty has increased most in rural counties of the US, and rural–urban differences in obesity are associated mostly with differences in education at the individual level, and economic and built environmental differences at the neighbourhood level. Obesity is also higher in counties of the US with the greatest population sprawl, where people spend much less time walking and more time in a motor car. While usually encouraging sedentary behaviour, the car can also enable positive values relating to food and physical activity (by increasing access to stores selling healthy food, and to resources for physical activity, such as the great outdoors), but more so for wealthier citizens than for poorer ones.

The built environment can shape physical activity patterns especially in ways that urban space is configured and organized, the types and organization of built and natural features (including architectural details and the quality of landscaping), transportation systems (especially the facilities and services that link one place to another), and environmental outputs from urban configurations and organization (including air quality, pollution, and perceptions of risk for personal safety).

Recognizing the structural issues that influence individual physical activity patterns, Adrian Bauman, at the University of Sydney, and his colleagues across the world, developed an ecological model of the determinants of physical activity, from the individual to the global and from early life to older age. Table 8.1 shows a multilayer framing of determinants of physical activity, which draws on the model of Bauman and colleagues. Much research in this area of study involves counting features that can be used in statistical analysis – food stores, pavements, parks – rather than how they are negotiated by people, reflecting an individualist bias. The framing given in Table 8.1 is most persuasive at the individual level, because there has been more research at this level than at interpersonal, environmental, state, regional, or global levels. Of individual-level factors, age, sex, health status, self-efficacy, and motivation have been identified as being positively associated with physical activity. At a higher level of organization, land-use mix, connectivity, population density, and overall neighbourhood design all influence individual physical activity. Walking as a form of transport, more than walking as a form of recreation, is perhaps the most important for maintaining health in the built environment, because this is the most regular form of physical activity taken.

Urban scale and shape matter for physical activity and obesity. Within cities of the US, compact areas have lower rates of obesity than sprawling ones, mostly because of differences in walkability and other possibilities for physical activity. Most of the larger conurbations in the US are now polycentric, following a global trend in urban growth across the past two decades or so. With polycentric urbanism, multiple independent centres have similar degrees of

Level	Factors influencing physical activity	Level of evidence	Policy responses
Individual	Behaviour and biology Evolution and genetics	Strong	Individualist
Interpersonal	Social support Norms and practices	Good	Community and social networks
Environmental	Social Built Natural	Acceptable	Socio-structural
State or regional	Transport systems Urban planning Sectors – parks, health, education, sports, corporate, advocacy groups	Weak	Structural
Global	Economic Urbanization Social and cultural	Speculative	Structural

Table 8.1   A multilayer framing of determinants of physical activity

importance, unlike monocentric cities, where there is a dominant centre. Jiawen Yang and Peiling Zhou, of Peking University and the Harbin Institute of Technology, Shenzhen, have shown, in an analysis of built environments in the US, that polycentric cities have lower obesity rates than monocentric or dispersed ones. They attribute the difference to differences in physical activity. In China, polycentric urban structures are more permissive of physical activity than are neighbourhood-level factors. Polycentric cities offer spatial variability of neighbourhood-level density, and of infrastructure such as street connectivity and land use mix, both of which promote physical activity and access to healthy food through efficient supply infrastructures. Lower obesity rates in polycentric cities may also be due to greater population densities, higher per-capita incomes, and lower poverty rates than monocentric or dispersed cities. Urban population concentration reduces dependence on the motor car and allows healthier eating through economies of scale in the distribution of healthy foods and higher local turnover of such foods (which often have short shelf-lives).

Research into neighbourhood effects on obesity shows two main features to dominate – the food environment and the physical activity environment. The food environment is considered in relation to physical access to food resources – especially supermarkets, grocery stores, fast food restaurants, and convenience stores. Physical activity environments are mostly seen in terms of area walkability, access to green and blue spaces, availability of recreational facilities, and land use mix. In neighbourhoods, walking, green space, active transport, and recreational facilities protect against obesity. Socioeconomic status is a more important correlate of obesity in neighbour-hoods than is physical proximity to food sources, whether these be supermar-kets or fast-food restaurants. People do only part of their business at the neighbourhood level, however, and commuting to work and mobility through car use for shopping and recreation make the neighbourhood a less-powerful shaper of behaviours related to obesity now than in the recent past, and especially since the rise of social media. One way in which positive neigh-bourhood-level health effects are being structurally put in place in some cities, is the 15-minute city idea of Carlos Moreno and colleagues at the Université Paris 1 Panthéon-Sorbonne. Taking as a starting point the knowledge that the quality of urban life is inversely proportional to the amount of time invested in transportation, especially with the use of motor cars, they have proposed urban set-ups where inhabitants are able to access all of their basic essentials within a 15-minute walk or cycle ride. This is seen as having many potential benefits by Moreno and colleagues, among them expected increases in phys-ical activity. Not everyone is sold on this idea, though. For example, car drivers in Oxford – and others with interests in having motorized access – are resisting a version of such a scheme, one that is approaching implementa-tion at the time of writing.

Within urban localities, domestic space has largely been left undisturbed by researchers of obesity and environment, except in relation to child-rearing and television use. A study of physical activity in the domestic space among young children in the US has revealed how this is related to family routine and activities of care, and to availability (or not) of domestic outside space, including yards and private gardens. The various lockdowns of the COVID-19 pandemic pushed public health firmly into the domestic arena, a domain of food and built environment research more usually linked to social psychology.

What Can We Do?

Some researchers have talked about there being an epidemic of sedentism, implicitly linking sitting down for long hours to chronic disease risk and obesity. Some media have gone so far as to say that sedentism 'is the new smoking'. That is probably over-stating the case for getting up and moving around more, but there is certainly some truth to it. We have evolved as a species to be physically active for much of the time. Our activity schedules are no longer linked to our dietary needs – most of us neither hunt nor gather, nor grow crops for our own consumption to any great extent, if at all. We now have physical inactivity schedules (as opposed to physical activity schedules) as our economic well-being is now more strongly linked to mental and cognitive activity, at least in wealthy countries. Much of the working population is shackled to the desk for long hours across most of the week, or engaged in work that is otherwise technologically mediated in some way. We need to be unshackled, or to unshackle ourselves from the devices that stop us being physically active, but how to do this? A start is to recognize that factors that influence physical activity vary across the life-course and to invoke different types of policy intervention, from individualist to social and structural approaches.

With respect to governmental policy aimed at increasing physical activity in the general population, implementation is difficult if workplaces require or privilege sedentism, and there are politically influential industries that promote the use of cars and forms of sedentary leisure. Urban planning has proved useful in engineering built environments that promote physical activity, as for example in Copenhagen. There, a five-finger plan of urban development was framed in 1947, which involved implementing a radiation of urban development from the centre of Copenhagen north and northeastwards along major train lines but which also encouraged active transport through the provision of cycle tracks, localized shopping, and local availability of other facilities. This was an early form of polycentricity, which we now know mitigates obesity through providing infrastructure and incentivizing active transport. More generally, walkability and active transport are both promoted widely in urban planning spheres. A common practice now is building in provision for cycling and walking, which both decongests cities of cars, and promotes physical and mental health and well-being, as well as offering some resistance to weight gain. Potential physical activity interventions at neighbourhood level are important, because if successful they are more likely to stick, because of the modelling of social norms within them. If everyone cycles, then cycling is what you do, even if you might not be as keen on it as the next person.

Current obesity control strategies often recommend increasing daily physical activity, with the assumption that increased activity will lead to corresponding increases in TEE, which in turn will promote healthy weight maintenance. However, according to Pontzer and colleagues, there is a ceiling on physical activity among people who are already active. The challenge is then to mobilize less physically active members of society to put on their running/walking/cycling shoes and move more. Another approach might be to promote NEAT. A NEAT approach to the workplace, for example, could promote physical activity among sedentary workers while at work. Since full-time work takes up around a half of most people's waking day, workstations that promote physical activity (even fidgeting) could help in maintaining healthy weight.

It is important to recognize just how much the structures of everyday life promote sedentism. Chairs and seating are everywhere, and while they are great to have, maybe we don't need to sit as much as we do. I have been at meetings in Copenhagen where people stand up for periods at a time because they are lethargic or fidgety from sitting. I have a Danish standing desk, which allows me to work while moving around on the spot – fidgeting – in the time-honoured way of authors like Ernest Hemingway, but also like many medieval scholars. At home, maybe we should spend less time on the sofa. Finding neat little ways to increase NEAT is a great way to increase energy expenditure.

Cycling to work is a productive form of NEAT because it is an everyday activity, but also a form of exercise.

Active transport is another way of increasing energy expenditure – cycling and walking are great for being engaged in the world around you while getting to work. Not all urban areas are blessed with appropriate or good facilities for either of these activities, and we should petition the authorities for more. Right now, the urban planners are listening, as they strive to improve the liveability of towns and cities. Using public transport rather than a car helps too – people who use a bus or a train to get to work are more physically active than those who do not, because they commonly walk to and from public transportation. After the COVID-19 pandemic, so many people continued to work from home for at least part of the week, making the promotion of physical activity in the domestic sphere all the more important. The built environment and the spaces within it influence levels of physical activity, although this is structured by strong sociodemographic factors. Perceived danger is a factor that can influence how and when (if at all) people walk in poor neighbourhoods. In the 1990s, I lived in a poor part of a big city in the US. While I felt intimidated to walk much in my neighbourhood, I also felt that riding a bicycle helped to keep me safe because I could avoid or cycle away from potentially dangerous situations. Similarly, my friend and colleague Sabine Parrish told me that she gained a lot of weight when in Sao Paulo, mostly because she lived somewhere where she didn't feel safe on the streets for much of the day, so she hardly walked or cycled. Cleaning up a neighbourhood and getting to know people can improve walkability by reducing perceptions of danger and risk.

Physical activity may not have much direct effect on body weight beyond keeping it stable, but it has indirect effects, like matching appetite to energy expenditure (Chapter 7), and contributing to healthy ways of life that include good diet, sociality, and regular engagement with open spaces. I couldn't do without all of these good things that physical activity brings – the amazing (and very open, socially) open-water swimming community I am part of, brings them all by the bucketful. You can know where to find me almost any early morning of the year, in or by the water in Oxford, Oxfordshire, or Hyde Park, London.

9 Making an Imperfect Storm

Between an Old Fashioned and a Manhattan

The first time I went to Japan, nearly three decades ago now, I took a short walk from my hotel near the University of Tokyo into the foggy and still night without a map, without the World Wide Web, without any knowledge of the Japanese language. It was November, a thick white blanket of almost frozen vapour covering everything outside, including my visual and mental perception. As my spectacles fogged up, adding another layer to my perceptual fogginess, I walked a hundred paces one way down the street then back again. Then another hundred in the other direction. Turning a corner to the left, then back again. Then two hundred in the other direction. You get the picture; I was building an image, a mind-map, of an unusually silent foggy island within the usually hustle-bustling city of Tokyo. When I felt I had done enough mental mapping I went back to my hotel room and drew a physical map on a scrap of paper of my walk. I have it somewhere still. I did something similar in Berlin the following year, 1995. The world was changing, Soviet-style socialism had collapsed and with it, so had the Berlin Wall. The physical map I had with me that day revealed no sign of it. I spent my only free afternoon there walking and retracing the Berlin Wall on my map from traces and remnants still to be found on the ground, if you looked for them. 'Die Mauer im Kopf' – the wall in the head – has continued to be there in Berlin. People there have no need to be reminded of the physical wall, they have a map of it in their minds. Mapping is first and foremost a mental process – mapping the unknown makes it knowable, even if imperfectly so. I have always been driven to understand the un-understandable, and maps are indispensable to this. Mapping obesity helps us to understand it. And understanding obesity takes many forms, none of which can be mobilized individually to control or regulate obesity – there is no menu to pick and choose from. But these different forms come together in different ways at different times and in different countries, creating an imperfect storm for the production of obesity. Why imperfect? If it were perfect, it would be the same everywhere, but it's not. There are so many pathways to obesity, at the individual and population level, that it beggars belief. It's a storm for sure, imperfectly different in every country and society.

When I talk about the many factors come together to create the imperfect storm of obesity, people still seek a single-factor explanation. I remember talking with Joy at a party, after the inevitable 'And what do you do?' question, which I detest, about obesity. I made the mistake of thinking she was genuinely interested, and spoke freely of its multifactorial nature, how different factors come together in different ways to create an imperfect storm for obesity, both individually and on a large scale. Just before turning and going our separate ways, she came back with 'What if it just turns out to be the microbiome?' (the latest new fad factor of that time). I let it go, my irritation with her, but thought, 'She hasn't listened to a word I said.' It gave me a new interpretation of the phrase 'a wall in the head' – a rigid and made-up mind – as well as giving me added motivation to write this book.

It's a pity that the party wasn't a cocktail party, but later I restaged the scene with Joy, in my mind's eye – at a cocktail party. I quite like the glamour of dressing up in order to stand around with a fancy drink, an Old Fashioned, in my hand and make idle conversation. In this fantasy cocktail party, I replied to Joy's last word by saying, 'That's a Manhattan in your glass, isn't it?' Then she paused, and I explained the cocktail that is obesity, by way of the cocktail in my own hand – an Old Fashioned. A Manhattan is more complicated to make than an Old Fashioned, while the imperfect storm that is obesity is downright complex. If you are partial to a cocktail, try drinking the ingredients of a Manhattan separately – bourbon whiskey, sweet vermouth, Angostura bitters, orange bitters. Each is distinctive, the latter two also being undrinkable neat, but the cocktail is both a mix of all of these ingredients and not like any of them at all, individually. So it is with obesity – each understanding about it is much more of a partial truth than a complete one. A complete understanding of obesity contains the understandings of all of the chapters of this book, but is not like any of them individually. Obesity is complex, more so than an Old Fashioned or a Manhattan, and its emergence in human societies has many properties of complexity – of having a tipping point where it all kicks off, then running away towards who knows where.

Can obesity be reversed? Should it be reversed? What should be done? What can be done? The literature on obesity interventions has a history of hollow claims and fake triumphalism. The media haven't helped, looking as they do for quick fixes and simple explanations. The logic of news reporting includes disseminating what is novel, what affects the public, and whether social institutions are effective in addressing public challenges. In relation to obesity, the media don't really help in any meaningful way, either in understanding why it has continued to rise in populations, or in knowing how you might best shape your life to avoid putting on weight or to take it off, if you already have excess weight. With that in mind, in this final chapter I discuss the cocktail of complexity that is obesity, the logic of media messaging in relation to body fatness and obesity, and in a summative way examine what can be done in governance and policy, and by individuals, to come to terms with obesity, body fatness and body weight respectively.

Obesity as Complexity

The first systematic attempt to frame obesity as a matter of complexity came in the early 2000s with the UK Government Foresight Obesities project. This process was about finding effective policy responses to this tricky problem, after a decade of policy failure. Foresight Obesities considered how over a hundred factors viewed to be associated with obesity worked together, bringing them together within one systems map. More has become known since then, but the mapping process employed by Foresight Obesities characterized the complexity of this phenomenon beyond simple description. This project sought to 'de-silo' obesity research and policy by bringing together very diverse stakeholders to the cause of obesity management and control. Reframing obesity as a complex problem requiring multiple sites of intervention, the project aimed to move responses to this issue away from personal responsibility and towards structural factors, like inequality and the production of what subsequently came to be known as ultra-processed foods (UPFs).

Although obesity had been described as being complex prior to Foresight Obesities, the vast majority of scholarly literature on obesity framed its complexity within discrete, siloed, domains of physiology, psychology, genetics, and treatment. A complex problem is one that involves multiple actors and factors connected to each other either directly or indirectly, such that it is impossible to anticipate the effect of a change in any single factor. This is quite different from a simple problem where the outcomes of actions are linear and can be predicted, and where interventions are also linear and can be predicted. This makes fixing obesity much more difficult than smoking and lung cancer, for example. If you were to say to someone, 'If you smoke, it will (eventually) kill you,' you would be much closer to the mark than if you said, 'If you eat too much you will develop obesity.' Possible causes of lung cancer are much closer to linearity than are possible causes of obesity. The tendency of everyday people, politicians, media, and health professionals to seek linear causation for obesity is a problem of framing that gets in the way of its understanding. It doesn't help that it is difficult to state the causes of obesity with any real confidence. At a recent meeting of experts at the Royal Society of London, one of the most august scientific bodies in the world, it was impossible to reach consensus on this matter, although there was consensus on the complexity of obesity production. Outside of the Royal Society and in everyday life, we are wedded to linear narratives, stories, even in a world where much cutting-edge fictional writing attempts to undermine or explode such linearity. While there is acknowledgement of the complexity of obesity among policymakers, at least in the UK, there is a long way to go with extending this understanding to everyday life, and the media don't help.

Obesity and the Media

When the Foresight obesity systems map was released, the media had a field day, subverting this new narrative about obesity. This is unsurprising – news media take a critical stance toward authority of any kind, including medical science, and especially politics. Given the dominant position of formal media in mediating between science, policy and citizens, the choice of many professionals to question obesity complexity before understanding it, has perpetuated many everyday misunderstandings about obesity, which are described at the end of this book. In 2013, the American Medical Association identified obesity as being a complex, chronic disease, but the public continued to consume a media narrative that views obesity to be largely one of individual control. With ongoing research, obesity has been ever more clearly defined as a complex, multifactorial disorder, with unique issues for each person with obesity, and with multiple pathways of its development (as with chronic diseases – see Chapters 1, 3, 4, and 8) among different local and national populations. So why do the media carry on reporting obesity as if nothing has changed in obesity science and policy?

For starters, obesity often gets cast as a form of moral deviance in media reporting, when stark words are deployed about the personal consequences of carrying excess body fat. Media representations also use obesity as a means of discussing themes society is uncomfortable with, as in the US, with poverty, race and/or ethnicity. Use by formal media of terms like 'obesity crisis' and 'obesity war' is a problem, too. In some countries (like the US and UK) people classified as being of normal body size according to their body mass index (BMI) are now in the minority, making a majority of the population morally deviant on this basis. Any 'war on obesity' becomes a war against moral deviants, those who are portrayed as being unable to take control of their lives – people who are fat, or poor, or Black, or women, or any combination of all of these – regardless of the structural issues that make their lives what they are.

The Fat Acceptance Movement rejects terms like 'overweight' and obese' because they medicalize fat bodies. Rather, the movement reclaims the term 'fat' in framing larger bodies as being part of natural and desirable diversity, alongside gender fluidity and ancestry. From its origins in 1967 as a sit-in protest of several hundred people in Central Park, New York City, the Fat Acceptance Movement has grown in parallel with the rise of obesity. Negative framings of obesity now alienate many people with excess weight, who no longer see themselves as minority deviants, who have alternative narratives of large body size to those offered by a largely unchanging formal media.

Media discourses in Western societies have largely privileged and validated the slender female body for over a century, with cultural beauty ideals rigidly emphasizing thinness for women. In general, more women across the world are likely to carry excess body weight than men. Especially in wealthy countries, slimness as a form of embodied cultural capital (Chapter 6) is sought by the majority of women. Idealized images of women in mass media influence how women view themselves. Although wealthier people in the UK are more concerned about body shape and are more likely to engage in efforts to lose weight than poorer people, women show more weight concern than do men, regardless of social and economic position. The scientific community often doesn't help, or can't help, the situation, especially where funding and professional advancement favour novelty, competition, and focused findings rather than complexity, mess, and debate. Scientific knowledge is almost always incomplete, especially at the cutting edge, when the role of scientists is to probe an issue through diverse methodologies to reveal solid truths about it. Science moves to consensus through data and debate, and most everyday science is not about consensus but about data. By focusing on novelty, media reporting of obesity science often creates a bias – something that confirms an earlier observation is simply not newsworthy, while something that refutes it might well be, thus making it seem like the scientists can't make up their minds. It is no surprise that public ideas about obesity are often confused and varied. In that these ideas become the basis for cultural judgements about body fatness and obesity, the media do not lie blameless in perpetuating stigma, blame, and moral judgement about body size and fatness. There are always beneficiaries to confusion, and the media earn many air miles by framing the complexity of obesity a mess, and calling the experts incompetent because they don't frame this complexity as simplicity.

People carrying excess weight get a rough deal. I can sit at the bar drinking my Imperfect Storm cocktail, reading the news media about obesity on my phone, or I can get out and do something. That something, for an obesity scientist, is to help shape the world in some small way, but in a good way. For me, that good way is to help people understand how the imperfect storm of obesity is created, to help people and policymakers act in more appropriate ways. So what can we really do?

What Can We Really Do?

Political arithmetic is a term I like, out-of-fashion though it is. It was coined in the seventeenth century by Sir William Petty, one of the founder members of the Royal Society, London, to describe the application of metrics to practical issues of governance. This practical science has since been subsumed within economics, with the term lapsing into disuse. With its metrics collected globally and applied to public health and personal well-being, and framed as risk in present-day risk society, the governance of obesity is to my view a form of political arithmetic, much more so than a tiny interest in the hold of the oil tanker that is economics. Governing obesity across the past three decades-plus has become a fraught enterprise, as the simple solutions, usually invoking personal responsibility, have ended in abject failure.

The starting point in any political discussion of obesity is with its metrics – how many people, where, how old, according to gender, according to race/ethnicity/ancestry. There is no measure of obesity that is collected nearly as systematically as the BMI. While over half of all nation-states collect population-level obesity rates at least once per decade, very few undertake data collection of any other anthropometric measures of obesity at this level. Epidemiological data collection and reporting, and the use of obesity epidemiology in econometric modelling of the impacts of obesity, are usually starting points for state-led obesity interventions. Obesity as a risk factor has been situated in framing health policy, because it sits among other risk categories such as smoking, unhealthy diet, and physical inactivity for chronic disease onset and progression. Categories of risk have ambivalent status in policymaking, however. For example, unhealthy diet is damaging, but the food industry, which is tasked with supplying uncontaminated and affordable food to large populations, primarily seeks to continue its operations without undue regulation. The spur to policy action by most nation-states is overwhelmingly economic, as the most persuasive political arguments usually involve framing obesity as a significant burden to the economy and the health service. This is generally measured through costs to employers, issues of medical management, and associated levels and trends in chronic diseases. If the data are not collected and/or mapped, then the problem cannot really be deemed to exist as a matter for policy. That said, comparing obesity rates across different countries needs to be done with caution, as the relationships between BMI, fatness, and disease vary across different populations. And if you get away from the BMI, the relationships with disease and death differ according to which measure of obesity is used, the population under investigation (be it of European, Asian, or African ancestry, young or old, male or female), and among the various classificatory boundaries that are used in obesity research and practice. So is all lost? I don't think so – there are many areas in life where it is possible to act on imperfect knowledge, and so it should be with the governance of obesity.

BMI is a measure that is just about good enough, no more no less, to be able to infer success or failure in anti-obesity policy and action. Despite this being the most widely used measure, other measures, like waist circumference and waist to height ratio, relate both to extent and type of body fat, and to risk of chronic disease, more strongly than the BMI. In the formalization of BMI for international use in the measurement of obesity and its correlates, the likelihood of obesity misclassification was acknowledged. It was deemed acceptable, however, given the overarching programmatic aim to provide simplicity for assessment and monitoring worldwide. So we continue to have an imperfect political arithmetic of obesity, where the measure used in governance is imperfect and clearly known to be so, and where it might be difficult now to seriously change the system of obesity reporting worldwide.

As we come to know more about genetics and genomics, could such data be incorporated into the political arithmetic of obesity? It is surely a matter of time, given that data is currency in present-day society, shaping our lives in so many ways. Genome-wide association studies with metabolomics (mGWAS) now reveal how interconnected the genetic regulation of energy metabolism is (Chapter 3). Adding such an approach to conventional epidemiology would add layers of complexity to understandings of obesity, with implications for its governance.

Good governance requires responsibility, accountability, awareness, impartiality, and transparency, all in good measure. While this set of principles does not operate cleanly in most countries, it is critically important as a set of ideals and aspirations. If governments struggle with achieving good governance, then maybe individuals can govern themselves better than governments can their countries? Perhaps to a degree, but it's actually very complicated. People need structural help to resist obesity. Amandine Garde, of the University of Liverpool, has advocated for legal and human rights-based approaches to work against obesogenic commercial practices. Human rights approaches to obesity have been taken up by the United Nations in treaty organizations (such as the United Nations Committee on Economic, Social and Cultural Rights), calling on nation-states to address risk factors for obesity under treaties that they have signed up to.

French sociologist Michel Foucault made it clear in his writings of the 1970s that governance extends to the self. If obesity is one outcome of living in an unequal society, then perhaps we have brought it on ourselves, through poor governance at every level, especially across the past four decades with the rise and normalization of neoliberalism and the neoliberal self. Helene Shugart, of the University of Utah, has described how popular discourses regarding obesity now often oppose governmental and corporate discourses of obesity (in relation to personal responsibility) which are seen in terms of failures of neoliberalism by many. Such discourses take several forms, including environmentalism, fatalism, emotional and/or spiritual dysfunction, resistance, cultural difference, and disgrace (of the self, of government, of corporations). We can challenge or acknowledge the damage that market economies do, as well as the good that they can create.

The political economic systems that especially favour neoliberalism have helped create obesogenic environments, and have helped make UPFs attractive drugs of choice among many seeking solace from the stresses of everyday life. At the national level, governments can regulate environments and food systems, and through taxation and social support can influence the extent of inequality in a nation. However, most anti-obesity interventions are neutral in respect of inequalities in obesity.

Public health intervention studies assume a level policy playing field, but this never really exists. For example, with respect to common obesity, a composite view of obesity genetics may be incorporated into public health responses to it, but minority groups would be left out. According to Kristin Young and colleagues at the University of North Carolina, minority populations which bear much of the obesity burden in the US have very low participation in genome-wide association studies (GWAS), including those related to obesity. In 2016, a mere 3 per cent of GWAS participants were of African ancestry, while people of South American/Hispanic ancestry were below 0.3 per cent of all GWAS participants. Another example lies with upstream structural interventions which could have the potential to improve the welfare of populations, which can be subverted by corporations, with world views that are governed by profit, and usually not welfare. Far-sighted governments might dare to go beyond being broadly popular and focus policy much more on maternal health and child-centred social investment. This would be economically expensive but socially productive, because it would help to reduce the legacy of obesity and chronic disease that has been created knowingly or not by past political, economic, social and colonial systems of power.

Obesity is personal as well as political. Most people can't put their body fatness down to having the wrong genetics or a slow metabolism, although those are likely to play some part. Obesity is complex, and we have to acknowledge this in relation to our own bodies and the ways in which we live our lives. Prudent ways of living, strong cognitive control of food intake both help, but we have to acknowledge the many forces against us when trying to eat healthily. Measurement can help too, in the political arithmetic of obesity policy and intervention, and to some extent for personal understanding. Most of us don't like to be thought of as a point on a chart, especially if that chart is one for our own BMI. If you are in the BMI grey zone (let's say between 25 and 30), then think also of how your body fat is distributed. This might be an unpleasant thought, given that most of us have some level of dissatisfaction with our bodies, but it's worth looking at ourselves naked in the mirror from time to time, and asking a few simple questions. 'Am I happy with what I see? Am I really fat? If I think I am, is my fatness on my hips, my belly, or my bum or my thighs?' If you think you carry excess body fat, you might be reassured if it's more on the hips, bum, or thighs than on the belly. If it's on the belly, then physical activity will help shape that up, along with avoiding alcohol, getting enough sleep, and avoiding stress. Being fit has a lot going for it, too. For example, people classified as being in the zone of normality for BMI, but unfit, have higher risk of dying from chronic disease than people also in the same BMI zone, but physically fit. For those of you who want to lose weight, the focus should not be solely placed on losing body weight or fatness, but also on increasing cardiorespiratory fitness, since even moderate fitness can reduce adverse health consequences of obesity. And if you're active, you have the virtue of knowing you are active and that this will help take fat out of your viscera and liver, both places where your body fat can do damage. But there are aspects of body fat distribution you can't really do that much about, related as they are to genetics. So this can only go so far, after which it is a matter of loving yourself and your body, however imperfect you feel you are.

Concluding Remarks

You know, you are not to blame if you put on excess body fatness, even if medical and political forces push it down on you. Generations of putting obesity onto individual responsibility reflects lazy politics and medical practice (or at least underestimating the complexity of the issue), not lazy people. Policy should help, not hinder, people's desire to be healthy at whatever size they feel good at. The free market, however, sets the backdrop for the drama associated with weight gain, body fatness, and obesity.

We are constantly persuaded by advertising, by the government, and formal media, that we can shape or identities and our destinies. This sounds very nice, but few of us are truly capable of doing so beyond a limited degree. Applying the rhetoric of choice to how we live our lives, to what and how we choose to eat, is great until you think about what is shaping our choices.

We can try to live less stressful lives – easier said than done, though. Or we can find ways of reducing stress that don't involve eating or any self-harming practice (like smoking, drinking alcohol, or use of illicit drugs). Physical activity, whatever that might involve, works for a lot of people. But even there, the physical structure of where you live might preclude exercise – you might live in suburbia with very limited public transport, or you might live a very urban life where the surroundings are physically dangerous or don't really support physical activity. Being critical of how life is shaped for you, rather than by you, is a good first step to working out just how much control of your circumstances is possible. Obesity for many people is an outcome of powerlessness, and even an inability to know how to act in present-day society. Often fixing one thing, seemingly unrelated to obesity, can help with weight control, especially if that one thing fixed reduces insecurity and uncertainty.

Most people I know have gone on a weight-loss diet at some time in their life. I have done so more than once. Most dieting and weight-loss approaches to obtaining and maintaining healthy weight make use of the energy balance model, with logic based in metabolism. They don't seem to work so well across longer time frames, giving only modest weight loss with either exercise or dietary restriction, and only slightly greater weight loss when exercise is combined with dietary restriction. This has led many researchers to challenge the usefulness of energy balance models as the basis for weight-loss interventions.

Other people don't help if they take a critical view of someone else's large body size. Medicine and science can take a lead, to avoid implicit stigma in their messaging. Currently, much of the world is questioning the historical supremacy of White people, with discourses of decolonization, and of de-stigmatization entering many fields. Intersectionalities – of race, of sex, of gender identity and sexual orientation, of disability – are all under scrutiny, and obesity science and intervention should strive to decolonize and remove stigma and blame from its practices. Social justice for people of excess weight should be a human right.

Maybe obesity might end with medication, if the promise of what is possible for those with extreme (usually monogenic) obesity can extend to the larger community of people carrying lower levels of excess weight. Or with sema-glutide, the drug designed for treatment of type 2 diabetes, now recruited to treatment of common obesity. The social scientist in me would urge caution. A number of questions spring to mind in response to the question 'What if the war on obesity were won tomorrow, with this new and effective medication?' For a start, who would decide who gets medication, and on what basis? And what would replace the stigma and (self) blame attached to obesity now? I suspect that the moralizing wouldn't stop, at least on the basis of what Karen Throsby, of the University of Leeds, has written about people undergoing bariatric surgery – 'Taking the easy way out' sums up the critical tone taken by some (non-overweight) people. Medication might fix obesity for some people, but we also have to decide how we want to live. When people stop their semaglutide injections, body fatness comes flooding back. Is that how we want to live with body fatness, with a yoyo of medicated weight loss followed by medication cessation and weight gain, then weight loss again with medication, and weight gain again after coming off it again? And again and again. Who knows what the long-term health implications of such behaviour might be?

Understanding obesity involves understanding complexity, of how the Imperfect Storm obesity cocktail is made up differently in different places and for different people. It also involves understanding ourselves. When we look in the mirror, what do we see? I, for one, fool myself into seeing a simple soul. The reality is that like obesity, we are all complex beings, and understanding obesity is also about seeing complexity in ourselves and in other people. And taking that understanding to the level of society – we are social beings, built to see and understand social complexity in its many forms. Looking at obesity in all these ways is a way of looking at how we live our lives. In the end, understanding obesity is perhaps more about understanding ourselves and others in the world now, than about fixing a problem.

Summary of Common Misunderstandings

Common misunderstandings about obesity as considered in this book are all correct understandings to some degree, but not in any total way. They include the following:

All body fat is bad. The truth of the matter is that the especially medically harmful fat is to be found inside your abdomen and around your gut, as well as in the liver. So many people have fatty livers in Western societies that it is not trivial. But physical activity helps burn metabolically harmful internal fat, around the gut and in the liver. Fat on the outside – subcutaneous fat – might be aesthetically displeasing to some, but doesn't carry nearly as much health risk. Fat on the bum and thighs, especially in women, is actually protective against chronic disease.

It's all due to my genes. Genetics is key to monogenic obesity but less so to common obesity, even though it plays an important part. Genetic expression is also hugely important, and the switching on or off of genetics linked to appetite and metabolism by environmental factors (mainly diet) especially so. Unless you carry extreme levels of body fat, it's unlikely to be down to genetics especially, and if it is, it is also down to expression of your genetics by environmental factors, especially diet, and of your mother's and grandmother's genetics.

It's all due to slow metabolism. Metabolism is important, but mostly not in terms of being either fast or slow, but in terms of being flexible. True, some people burn more energy and can eat all they want and not put on weight, while others cannot, but the vast majority of people are along a continuum of metabolic rate between either extreme. But regardless of where you sit on the continuum, your metabolism has evolved to protect you against weight loss, which would have been a key adaptation to survival in the past, but not so now, in times of food plenty. Trying to lose excess body weight is hard.

The food corporations are to blame. Ultra-processed foods made by companies big and small are damaging to health and help promote body fat gain. These foods are made with profit and shareholder value in mind, not health. You might feel good while you eat them, but they slowly corrode your body. They are everywhere, and while regulating their promotion and sale is underway in many countries, this still has a long way to go. If your body and your health are important to you, make a mental check of all the places you might encounter UPFs, which is a lot. And try to avoid places and circumstances where you might be tempted, because they are made to be tempting.

Society is to blame. Inequality and insecurity are bad for obesity, and stigma makes it worse. The free-market-based, neoliberal world we live in now needs inequality to be able to be in business. The stresses of living in neoliberal societies, with their multiple insecurities, are unlikely to disappear any time soon, because neoliberalism is not going away any time soon. What you can do though is to be aware, be a good person, fight against injustice, bodily, dietary, and of all other kinds.

You've only got yourself to blame. The odds are stacked against you if you want to lose weight, and this goes for everyone. Bodily stigma and blame are widespread in everyday life, even though medical institutions are trying to do something about it. Be self-compassionate about your own body fatness (if that is a concern for you) and compassionate about that of others. Don't blame them for the weight they carry, it might just be an outward sign of the hidden burdens they carry in life.

You eat too much. Most of us can eat too much if the circumstances favour it. We have evolved with a predisposition to do so. We can very easily overeat relative to our needs on a regular basis if we make UPFs our go-to foods. Some people have no choice – they can't afford or can't locate healthy foods locally, and UPFs are cheap, and everywhere. Be compassionate about other people's food and eating issues.

You don't get enough physical activity. Physical activity can help match appetite to calorie intake and help maintain a healthy weight, but on its own, it is not a way to lose weight. However, it is a great way to get to feel good about yourself, and maintain good mental as well as physical health. Take a walk, take a run, go for a swim, preferably outdoors – green and blue spaces are good for us, increasing evidence tells us.

Obesity is simple. No it's not. If it were, it would have been fixed decades ago. Obesity is complex, with many ingredients, in an imperfect storm. That's why its causes are varied and different, according to context – time of life, which country you live in, where you live within a country, where you seem to be placed in society. Look at your life and work out where the obesity triggers are, and there are many. Your triggers won't be someone else's, but they are as complex as the next person's.

References and Further Reading

Chapter 1

Blüher, M. (2020). Metabolically healthy obesity. *Endocrine Reviews* 41: bnaa004.

Bray, G. (2004). Medical consequences of obesity. *Journal of Clinical Endocrinology and Metabolism* 89: 2583–2589.

de Vries, J. (2007). The obesity epidemic: medical and ethical considerations. *Science and Engineering Ethics* 13: 55–67.

Doll, H. A., Peterson, S. E. K. & Stewart-Brown, S. L. (2000). Obesity and physical and emotional well-being: associations between body mass index, chronic illness, and the physical and mental components of the SF-36 questionnaire. *Obesity Research* 8: 160–170.

Jih, J., Mukherjea, A., Vittinghoff, E., Nguyen, T. T. et al. (2014). Using appropriate body mass index cut points for overweight and obesity among Asian Americans. *Preventive Medicine* 65: 1–6.

King, N. A., Hills, A. P. & Blundell, J. E. (2005). High body mass index is not a barrier to physical activity: analysis of international rugby players' anthropometric data. *European Journal of Sport Science* 5: 73–75.

Komlos, J. & Baur, M. (2004). From the tallest to (one of) the fattest: the enigmatic fate of the American population in the 20th century. *Economics & Human Biology* 2: 57–74.

Otero, M., Lago, R., Lago, F. et al. (2005). Leptin, from fat to inflammation: old questions and new insights. *FEBS Letters* 579: 295–301.

Prospective Studies Collaboration (2009). Body-mass index and cause-specific mortality in 900 000 adults: collaborative analyses of 57 prospective studies. *The Lancet* 373: 1083–1096.

Saito, M., Matsushita, M., Yoneshiro, T. & Okamatsu-Ogura, Y. (2020). Brown adipose tissue, diet-induced thermogenesis, and thermogenic food ingredients: from mice to men. *Frontiers in Endocrinology* 11: 222.

Thomas, E. L., Parkinson, J. R., Frost, G. S. et al. (2012). The missing risk: MRI and MRS phenotyping of abdominal adiposity and ectopic fat. *Obesity* 20: 76–87.

Ulijaszek, S. J. & McLennan, A. K. (2016). Framing obesity in UK policy from the Blair years, 1997–2015: the persistence of individualistic approaches despite overwhelming evidence of societal and economic factors, and the need for collective responsibility. *Obesity Reviews* 17: 397–411.

van der Klaauw, A. A., Horner, E. C., Pereyra-Gerber, P. et al. (2023). Accelerated waning of the humoral response to COVID-19 vaccines in obesity. *Nature Medicine* 29: 1146–1154.

Walker, G. E., Verti, B., Marzullo, P. et al. (2007). Deep subcutaneous adipose tissue: a distinct abdominal adipose depot. *Obesity* 15: 1933–1943.

World Health Organization (2000). *Obesity: Preventing and Managing the Global Epidemic*. Report of a WHO Consultation. Geneva: World Health Organization.

World Health Organization (2009). *Global Health Risks: Mortality and Burden of Disease Attributable to Selected Major Risks*. Geneva: World Health Organization.

World Health Organization (2014). *Ten Facts about Obesity*. Geneva: World Health Organization.

Wright, E. J. & Whitehead, T. L. (1987). Perceptions of body size and obesity: a selected review of the literature. *Journal of Community Health* 12: 117–129.

Chapter 2

Allison, D. B., Kaprio, J., Korkeila, M. et al. (1996). The heritability of body mass index among an international sample of monozygotic twins reared apart. *International Journal of Obesity and Related Metabolic Disorders* 20: 501–506.

Barker, D. J. P. (1995). Fetal origins of coronary heart disease. *BMJ* 311: 171–174.

Drong, A. W., Lindgren, C. M. & McCarthy, M. I. (2012). The genetic and epigenetic basis of type 2 diabetes and obesity. *Clinical Pharmacology and Therapeutics*, https://doi.org/10.1038/clpt.2012.149

Frayling, T. M., Timpson, N. J., Weedon, M. N. et al. (2007). A common variant in the FTO gene is associated with body mass index and predisposes to childhood and adult obesity. *Science* 316: 889–894.

Hall, K. D., Farooqi, I. S., Friedman, J. M. et al. 2022. The energy balance model of obesity: beyond calories in, calories out. *American Journal of Clinical Nutrition* 115: 1243–1254, https://doi.org/10.1093/ajcn/nqac031

Helgeland, O., Sole-Navais, P., Flatley, C. et al. (2022). Characterization of the genetic architecture of infant and early childhood body mass index. *Nature Metabolism* 4: 344–358.

Hofker, M. & Wijmenga, C. (2009). A supersized list of obesity genes. *Nature Genetics* 41: 139–140.

Johannsen, W. (1909). *Elemente der exakten Erblich-keitslehre*. Jena: Gustav Fischer.

Kimura, M. (1983). *The Neutral Theory of Molecular Evolution*. Cambridge: Cambridge University Press.

Loos, R. J. & Yeo, G. S. (2022). The genetics of obesity: from discovery to biology. *Nature Reviews Genetics* 23: 120–133.

Neel, J. (1962). Diabetes mellitus: a 'thrifty' genotype rendered detrimental by 'progress'? *American Journal of Human Genetics* 14: 353–362.

Patel, P., Babu, J. R., Wang, X. & Geetha, T. (2022). Role of macronutrient intake in the epigenetics of obesity. *Biochemical Society Transactions* 50: 487–497, https://doi.org/10.1042/BST20211069

Ravelli, A., van der Meulen, J., Osmond, C., Barker, D. & Bleker, O. (1999). Obesity at the age of 50 y in men and women exposed to famine prenatally. *American Journal of Clinical Nutrition* 70: 811–816, https://doi.org/10.1093/ajcn/70.5.811

Rutter, H. (2011). Where next for obesity? *Lancet* 378: 746–747.

Sellayah, D., Cagampang, F. R. & Cox, R. D. (2014). On the evolutionary origins of obesity: a new hypothesis. *Endocrinology* 155: 1573–1588.

Sørensen, T. I., Price, R. A., Stunkard, A. J. & Schulsinger, F. (1989). Genetics of obesity in adult adoptees and their biological siblings. *British Medical Journal* 298: 87–90.

Speakman, J. R. (2007). A nonadaptive scenario explaining the genetic predisposition to obesity: the 'predation release' hypothesis. *Cell Metabolism* 6: 5–12.

Speakman, J. R. (2008). Thrifty genes for obesity, an attractive but flawed idea, and an alternative perspective: the 'drifty gene' hypothesis. *International Journal of Obesity* 32: 1611–1617.

von Noorden, C. (1907). *Metabolism and Practical Medicine*. Chicago: W. T. Keener and Company.

Yang, J., Manolio, T. A., Pasquale, L. R. et al. (2011). Genome partitioning of genetic variation for complex traits using common SNPs. *Nature Genetics* 43: 519–525.

Chapter 3

Abbots, E.-J., Eli, K. & Ulijaszek, S. (2020). Toward an affective political ecology of obesity mediating biological and social aspects. *Cultural Politics* 16: 346–366.

Berthoud, H. R. & Morrison, C. (2008). The brain, appetite, and obesity. *Annual Review of Psychology* 59: 55–92.

Carreiro, A. L., Dhillon, J., Gordon, S. et al. (2016). The macronutrients, appetite, and energy intake. *Annual Review of Nutrition* 36: 73–103.

Franz, M. J., van Wormer, J. J., Crain, A. L. et al. (2007). Weight-loss outcomes: a systematic review and meta-analysis of weight-loss clinical trials with a minimum 1-year follow-up. *Journal of the American Dietetic Association* 107: 1755–1767.

Frayn, K. (2022). *Understanding Metabolism*. Cambridge: Cambridge University Press.

Guyenet, S. J. & Schwartz, M. W. (2012). Regulation of food intake, energy balance, and body fat mass: implications for the pathogenesis and treatment of obesity. *Journal of Clinical Endocrinology and Metabolism* 97: 745–755.

Hall, K. D., Ludwig, D. S., Aronne, L. J. et al. (2021). The carbohydrate–insulin model: a physiological perspective on the obesity pandemic. *American Journal of Clinical Nutrition* 114: 1873–1885.

Kastenmuller, G., Raffler, J., Gieger, C. & Suhre, K. (2019). Genetics of human metabolism: an update. *Nutrients* 11: 1812, https://doi.org/10.3390/nu11081812

Ludwig, D. S. & Sørensen, T. I. (2022). An integrated model of obesity pathogenesis that revisits causal direction. *Nature Reviews Endocrinology* 18: 261–262.

Mayer, J. (1954). Glucostatic mechanism of regulation of food intake. *New England Journal of Medicine* 249: 13–16.

Saito, M., Okamatsu-Ogura, Y., Matsushita, M. et al. (2009). High incidence of metabolically active brown adipose tissue in healthy adult humans: effects of cold exposure and adiposity. *Diabetes* 58: 1526–1531.

Sellayah, D., Cagampang, F. R. & Cox, R. D. (2014). On the evolutionary origins of obesity: a new hypothesis. *Endocrinology* 155: 1573–1588.

Simpson, S. J. & Raubenheimer, D. (2005). Obesity: the protein leverage hypothesis. *Obesity Reviews* 6: 133–142.

Suzuki, K., Jayasena, C. N. & Bloom, S. R. (2011). The gut hormones in appetite regulation. *Journal of Obesity* 528401, https://doi.org/10.1155/2011/528401

Tun, H. M., Konya, T., Brook, J. R. et al. (2017). Exposure to household furry pets influences the gut microbiota of infants at 3–4 months following various birth scenarios. *Microbiome* 5: 1–14.

Ulijaszek, S. J. & Bryant, E. J. (2016). Binge eating, disinhibition and obesity. In *Evolutionary Thinking in Medicine: From Research to Policy and Practice* (ed. A. Alvergne, C. Jenkinson and C. Faurie) pp. 105–117. New York: Springer Publishing Company.

Zhenhua, L., Lingbing, M., Zhen, S. et al. (2021). Differentially expressed genes and enriched signaling pathways in the adipose tissue of obese people. *Frontiers in Genetics* 12: 2021, https://doi.org/10.3389/fgene.2021.620740

Chapter 4

Bates, S., Reeve, B. & Trevena, H. (2020). A narrative review of online food delivery in Australia: Challenges and opportunities for public health nutrition policy. *Public Health Nutrition* 26: 262–272.

Brice, J. P. (2021). The regulation of digital food platforms in the UK. *Food Law and Policy* 2: 53–106.

Centers for Disease Control (2017). Healthy Places – Healthy Food – General Food Environment Resources. www.cdc.gov. Retrieved 20 January 2023.

Cohen, D. (2008). Neurophysiological pathways to obesity: below awareness and beyond individual control. *Diabetes* 57: 1768–1773.

Di Nicolantonio, J. J., O'Keefe, J. H. & Wilson, W. L. (2018). Sugar addiction: is it real? A narrative review. *British Journal of Sports Medicine 52*: 910–913.

Downs, S. M., Ahmed, S., Fanzo, J. & Herforth, A. (2020). Food environment typology: advancing an expanded definition, framework, and methodological approach for improved characterization of wild, cultivated, and built food environments toward sustainable diets. *Foods* 9: 532, https://doi.org/10.3390/foods9040532

Elizabeth, L., Machado, P., Zinocker, M. et al. (2020). Ultra-processed foods and health outcomes: a narrative review. *Nutrients* 12: 1955, https://doi.org/10.3390/nu12071955

Fernandez, M. A. & Raine, K. D. (2019). Insights on the influence of sugar taxes on obesity prevention efforts. *Current Nutrition Reports* 8: 333–339.

Gibney, M. J. (2019). Ultra-processed foods: definitions and policy issues. *Current Developments in Nutrition* 3: nzy077.

Goran, M. & Ventura, E. E. (2020). *Sugarproof*. London: Penguin.

Lang, T. & Rayner, G. 2007. *Ecological Public Health*. Abingdon: Routledge.

Monteiro, C. A., Bertazzi, R., Levy, R. et al. (2010). Uma nova classificação de alimentos baseada na extensão e propósito do seu processamento. *Cadernos de Saúde Pública* 26, https://doi.org/10.1590/S0102-311X2010001100005

Monteiro, C. A., Cannon, G., Levy, R. B. et al. (2019). Ultra-processed foods: what they are and how to identify them. *Public Health Nutrition* 22: 936–941.

NCD Risk Factor Collaboration (NCD-RisC). (2019). Rising rural body-mass index is the main driver of the global obesity epidemic in adults. *Nature* 569: 260–264, https://doi.org/10.1038/s41586-019-1171-x

Paula Neto, H. A., Ausina, P., Gomez, L. S. et al. (2017). Effects of food additives on immune cells as contributors to body weight gain and immune-mediated metabolic dysregulation. *Frontiers in Immunology* 8: 1478.

Popkin, B. M. (2001). The nutrition transition and obesity in the developing world. *Journal of Nutrition* 131: 871S–873S.

Schneider, T., Eli, K., Dolan, C. & Ulijaszek, S. (eds.) (2018). *Digital Food Activism*. Routledge: London.

Swinburn, B., Egger, G. & Raza, F. (1999). Dissecting obesogenic environments: the development and application of a framework for identifying and prioritizing environmental interventions for obesity. *Preventive Medicine* 29: 563–570.

Turner, C., Aggarwal, A., Walls, H. et al. (2018). Concepts and critical perspectives for food environment research: a global framework with implications for action in low- and middle-income countries. *Global Food Security* 18: 93–101.

Ulijaszek, S. J. (2023). Obesity and environments external to the body. *Philosophical Transactions of the Royal Society of London, Series B*, https://doi.org/10.1098/rstb.2022.0226

Yudkin, J. (1972). *Pure, White and Deadly*. London: Davis-Poynter.

Chapter 5

Bambra, C. F., Hillier, F., Cairns, J. et al. (2015). How effective are interventions at reducing socioeconomic inequalities in obesity among children and adults? Two systematic reviews. *Public Health Research* 3: 1, https://doi.org/10.3310/phr03010

Baudrillard, J. (1970). *The Consumer Society: Myths and Structures*. New York, NY: Sage Publications.

Bourdieu, P. (1986). The forms of capital. In *Cultural Theory: An Anthology* 1 (ed. T. Kaposy and I. Szeman) pp. 81–93. Wiley.

Bratanova, B., Loughnan, S., Klein, O. et al. (2016). Poverty, inequality, and increased consumption of high calorie food: experimental evidence for a causal link. *Appetite* 100: 162–171.

Butland, B., Jebb, S., Kopelman, P. et al. (2007). *Tackling Obesities: Future Choices – Project Report*, 2nd edn. London: Foresight Programme of the Government Office for Science.

Esping-Andersen, G. (2002). A child-centred social investment strategy. In *Why We Need a New Welfare State* (ed. G. Esping-Andersen) pp. 26–68. Oxford: Oxford University Press.

Friel, S., Chopra, M. & Satcher, D. (2007). Unequal weight: equity oriented policy responses to the global obesity epidemic. *British Medical Journal* 335: 1241.

Hacker, J. S. (2019). *The Great Risk Shift: The New Economic Insecurity and the Decline of the American Dream*. Oxford University Press.

Kanter, R. & Caballero, B. (2012). Global gender disparities in obesity: a review. *Advances in Nutrition* 3: 491–498, https://doi.org/10.3945/an.112.002063

Marmot, M., Atkinson, T., Bell, J. et al. (2010). *Fair Society, Healthy Lives: Strategic Review of Health Inequalities in England – the Marmot Review*. London: Institute of Health Equity, University College London.

McLaren, L. (2007). Socioeconomic status and obesity. *Epidemiologic Reviews* 29: 29–48.

Offer, A., Pechey, R. & Ulijaszek, S. (2010). Obesity under affluence varies by welfare regimes: the effect of fast food, insecurity, and inequality. *Economics & Human Biology* 8: 297–308.

Schrecker, T. & Bambra, C. (2015). *How Politics Makes Us Sick: Neoliberal Epidemics*. London: Palgrave MacMillan.

Trentmann, F. (2007). Citizenship and consumption. *Journal of Consumer Culture* 7: 147–58.

Ulijaszek, S. J. (2012). Socio-economic status, forms of capital and obesity. *Journal of Gastrointestinal Cancer* 43: 3–7.

Ulijaszek, S. J. & McLennan, A. K. (2016). Framing obesity in UK policy from the Blair years, 1997–2015: the persistence of individualistic approaches despite overwhelming evidence of societal and economic factors, and the need for collective responsibility. *Obesity Reviews* 17: 397–411.

Vassallo, S. (2020). *Neoliberal Selfhood*. Cambridge University Press.

Chapter 6

Bodirsky, M. & Johnson, J. (2008). Decolonizing diet: healing by reclaiming traditional Indigenous foodways. *Cuizine: The Journal of Canadian Food Cultures/ Cuizine: Revue des cultures culinaires au Canada*, https://doi.org/10.7202/019373ar

Brewis, A. A. (2014). Stigma and the perpetuation of obesity. *Social Science & Medicine* 118: 152–158.

Brewis, A. A., Wutich, A., Falletta-Cowden, A. & Rodriguez-Soto, I. (2011). Body norms and fat stigma in global perspective. *Current Anthropology* 52: 269–276.

Chang, V. W. & Christakis, N. A. (2003). Self-perception of weight appropriateness in the United States. *American Journal of Preventive Medicine* 24: 332–339.

Chou, W. S., Prestin, A. & Kunath S. (2014). Obesity in social media: a mixed methods analysis. *Translational Behavioral Medicine* 4: 314–323.

Christakis, N. A. & Fowler, J. H. (2007). The spread of obesity in a large social network over 32 years. *New England Journal of Medicine* 357: 370–379.

Furedi, F. (2021). The diseasing of judgement: Frank Furedi chronicles the unravelling of moral authority. *First Things: A Monthly Journal of Religion and Public Life* 309: 31–37.

Jeon, Y. A., Hale, B., Knackmuhs, E. & Mackert, M. (2018). Weight stigma goes viral on the internet: systematic assessment of YouTube comments attacking overweight men and women. *Interactive Journal of Medical Research* 7: e9182.

Marcus, S.-R. (2016). Thinspiration vs. thicksperation: Comparing pro-anorexic and fat acceptance image posts on a photo-sharing site. *Cyberpsychology: Journal of Psychosocial Research on Cyberspace* 10: Article 5, https://doi.org/10.5817/CP2016-2-5

Millward, D. J. (2013). Energy balance and obesity: a UK perspective on the gluttony v. sloth debate. *Nutrition Research Reviews* 26: 89–109.

Monaghan, L. F., Colls, R. & Evans, B. (2013). Obesity discourse and fat politics: research, critique and interventions. *Critical Public Health* 23: 249–262.

Puhl, R. M. & Heuer, C. A. (2010). Obesity stigma: important considerations for public health. *American Journal of Public Health* 100: 1019–1028.

Rubino, F., Puhl, R. M., Cummings, D. E. et al. (2020). Joint international consensus statement for ending stigma of obesity. *Nature Medicine* 26: 485–497.

Schag, K., Schönleber, J., Teufel, M., Zipfel, S. & Giel, K. E. (2013). Food-related impulsivity in obesity and Binge Eating Disorder – a systematic review. *Obesity Reviews* 14: 477–495.

Shugart, H. A. (2016). *Heavy: The Obesity Crisis in Cultural Context.* Oxford: Oxford University Press.

Strings, S. (2019). *Fearing the Black Body. The Racial Origins of Fat Phobia.* New York: New York University Press.

Stryker, K. (2016). 6 Ways I Was Taught to Be a Good Fatty (And Why I Stopped). Blog Post in Everyday Feminism. https://everydayfeminism.com/2016/04/taught-to-be-good-fatty/

Tomiyama, A. J. (2014). Weight stigma is stressful. A review of evidence for the cyclic obesity/weight-based stigma model. *Appetite* 82: 8–15.

Ulijaszek, S. J., Mann, N. & Elton, S. (2012). *Evolving Human Nutrition: Implications for Public Health.* Cambridge: Cambridge University Press.

White, F. R. (2013). 'We're kind of devolving': visual tropes of evolution in obesity discourse. *Critical Public Health* 23: 320–330, https://doi.org/10.1080/09581596.2013.777693

Williams, O. & Annandale, E. (2019). Weight bias internalization as an embodied process: understanding how obesity stigma gets under the skin. *Frontiers in Psychology* 10: 953.

Williams, O. & Annandale, E. (2020). Obesity, stigma and reflexive embodiment: feeling the 'weight' of expectation. *Health* 24: 421–441.

Chapter 7

Angelidi, A. M., Belanger, M. J., Kokkinos, A., Koliaki, C. C. & Mantzoros, C. S. (2022). Novel noninvasive approaches to the treatment of obesity: from pharmacotherapy to gene therapy. *Endocrine Reviews* 43: 507–557.

Atwater, W. O. (1910). *Principles of Nutrition and Nutritive Value of Food* (No. 142). US Department of Agriculture.

Bergmann, N. C., Davies, M. J., Lingvay, I. & Knop, F. K. (2023). Semaglutide for the treatment of overweight and obesity: a review. *Diabetes, Obesity and Metabolism* 25: 18–35.

DiNicolantonio, J. J., O'Keefe, J. H. & Wilson, W. L. (2018). Sugar addiction: is it real? A narrative review. *British Journal of Sports Medicine* 52: 910–913.

Food and Agriculture Organization of the United Nations (2023). Food and Agriculture Data, https://www.fao.org/faostat/en/#home

Fukuyama, F. (1992). *The End of History and the Last Man*. New York: Simon and Schuster.

Herrick, C. (2009). Shifting blame/selling health: corporate social responsibility in the age of obesity. *Sociology of Health and Illness* 31: 51–65.

Ludwig, D. S. & Ebbeling, C. B. (2018). The carbohydrate-insulin model of obesity: beyond "calories in, calories out". *JAMA Internal Medicine* 178: 1098–1103.

Mejova, Y., Haddadi, H., Noulas, A. & Weber, I. (2015). #Foodporn: Obesity patterns in culinary interactions. In *Proceedings of the 5th International Conference on Digital Health 2015*, pp. 51–58.

Nguyen, P. K., Lin, S. & Heidenreich, P. (2016). A systematic comparison of sugar content in low-fat vs regular versions of food. *Nutrition and Diabetes* 6: e163.

Ochs, E. & Izquierdo, C. (2009). Responsibility in childhood: three developmental trajectories. *Ethos* 37: 391–413.

Petty, S., Salame, C., Mennella, J. A., & Pepino, M. Y. (2020). Relationships between taste detection thresholds and preference for sucrose in children, adolescents and adults. *Nutrients* 12: E1918.

Stubbs, R. J., Mazlan, N. & Whybrow, S. (2001). Carbohydrates, appetite and feeding behavior in humans. *Journal of Nutrition* 131: 2775S–2781S.

White, M., Aguirre, E., Finegood, D. T. et al. (2020). What role should the commercial food system play in promoting health through better diet? *BMJ* 368, https://doi.org/10.1136/bmj.m545

Wilding, J. P., Batterham, R. L., Davies, M. et al. & STEP 1 Study Group (2022). Weight regain and cardiometabolic effects after withdrawal of semaglutide: the STEP 1 trial extension. *Diabetes, Obesity and Metabolism* 24: 1553–1564.

Chapter 8

Bauman, A. E., Reis, R. S., Sallis, J. F. et al. (2012). Correlates of physical activity: why are some people physically active and others not? *Lancet* 380: 258–271.

Burini, R. C., Anderson, E., Durstine, J. L. & Carson J. A. (2020). Inflammation, physical activity, and chronic disease: an evolutionary perspective. *Sports Medicine and Health Science* 1: 1–6.

Chin, S. H., Kahathuduwa, C. N. & Binks, M. (2016). Physical activity and obesity: what we know and what we need to know. *Obesity Reviews* 17: 1226–1244.

Colman, E. (1998). Obesity in the Paleolithic era? The Venus of Willendorf. *Endocrine Practice* 4: 58.

Keys, A., Brozek, J., Henschel, A. et al. (1950). *The Biology of Human Starvation.* Minneapolis: University of Minnesota Press.

Kohl, H. W., Craig, C. L., Lambert, E. V. et al. (2012). The pandemic of physical inactivity: global action for public health. *Lancet* 380: 294–305.

Levine, J. A. (2023). The Fidget Factor and the obesity paradox. How small movements have big impact. *Frontiers in Sports and Active Living* 5: 1122938.

Malina, R. M. & Little, B. B. (2008). Physical activity: the present in the context of the past. *American Journal of Human Biology* 20: 373–391.

Moreno, C., Allam, Z., Chabaud, D., Gall, C. & Pratlong, F. (2021). Introducing the '15-Minute City': Sustainability, resilience and place identity in future post-pandemic cities. *Smart Cities* 4: 93–111.

NCD Risk Factor Collaboration (NCD-RisC). (2019). Rising rural body-mass index is the main driver of the global obesity epidemic in adults. *Nature* 569: 260–264, https://doi.org/10.1038/s41586-019-1171-x

Ortega, F. B., Ruiz, J. R., Labayen, I., Lavie, C. J. & Blair, S. N. (2018). The fat but fit paradox: what we know and don't know about it. *British Journal of Sports Medicine* 52: 151–153.

Parrish, S., Lavis, A., Potter, C. M. et al. (2022). How active can preschoolers be at home? Parents' and grandparents' perceptions of children's day-to-day activity, with implications for physical activity policy. *Social Science & Medicine* 292: 114557.

Pontzer, H., Durazo-Arvizu, R., Dugas, L. R. et al. (2016). Constrained total energy expenditure and metabolic adaptation to physical activity in adult humans. *Current Biology* 26: 410–417.

Potter, C., Parrish, S., Eli, K. et al. (2020). Changes in mental health, eating and physical activity in England across COVID-19 pandemic lockdown. *COVID-19 Insight Report #1*. Oxford: Unit for BioCultural Variation and Obesity.

Ulijaszek, S. J. (2007). Obesity, a disorder of convenience. *Obesity Reviews* 8: 183–187.

Ulijaszek, S. J. (2018). Physical activity and the human body in the (increasingly smart) built environment. *Obesity Reviews* 19: 84–93.

Yang, J. & Zhou, P. (2020). The obesity epidemic and the metropolitan-scale built environment: examining the health effects of polycentric development. *Urban Studies* 57: 39–55.

Chapter 9

Afful, A. A. & Ricciardelli, R. (2015). Shaping the online fat acceptance movement: talking about body image and beauty standards. *Journal of Gender Studies* 24: 453–472.

Butland, B., Jebb, S., Kopelman, P. et al. (2007). *Tackling Obesities: Future Choices – Project Report*, 2nd edn. London: Foresight Programme of the Government Office for Science.

Eli, K. & Ulijaszek, S. J. (eds.) (2014). *Obesity, Eating Disorders and the Media*. Farnham, Surrey: Ashgate Publishing.

Garde, A., Curtis, J. & De Schutter, O. (eds.) (2020). *Ending Childhood Obesity: A Challenge at the Crossroads of International Economic and Human Rights Law*. Edward Elgar Publishing.

Haqq, A. M., Chung, W. K., Dollfus, H. et al. (2022). Efficacy and safety of setmelanotide, a melanocortin-4 receptor agonist, in patients with Bardet-Biedl syndrome and Alström syndrome: a multicentre, randomised, double-blind, placebo-controlled, phase 3 trial with an open-label period. *The Lancet Diabetes & Endocrinology* 10: 859–868.

O'Hara, L. & Gregg, J. (2012). Human rights casualties from the 'war on obesity': why focusing on body weight is inconsistent with a human rights approach to health. *Fat Studies* 1: 32–46, https://doi.org/10.1080/21604851.2012.627790

Rich, E. (2011). 'I see her being obesed!': public pedagogy, reality media and the obesity crisis. *Health* 15: 3–21.

Shugart, H. (2016). *Heavy. The Obesity Crisis in Cultural Context*. Oxford: Oxford University Press.

Stanford, F. C., Tauqeer, Z. & Kyle, T. K. (2018). Media and its influence on obesity. *Current Obesity Reports* 7: 186–192.

Throsby, K. (2009). The war on obesity as a moral project: weight loss drugs, obesity surgery and negotiating failure. *Science as Culture* 18: 201–216.

Ulijaszek, S. J. (2015). With the benefit of foresight: obesity, complexity and joined-up government. *BioSocieties* 10: 213–228.

Ulijaszek, S. J. (2017). *Models of Obesity*. Cambridge: Cambridge University Press.

Ulijaszek, S. J. & McLennan, A. K. (2016). Framing obesity in UK policy from the Blair years, 1997–2015: the persistence of individualistic approaches despite overwhelming evidence of societal and economic factors, and the need for collective responsibility. *Obesity Reviews* 17: 397–411.

Young, K. L., Graff, M., Fernandez-Rhodes, L. & North, K. E. (2018). Genetics of obesity in diverse populations. *Current Diabetes Reports* 18: 145.

Figure Credits

Index

Locators in *italic* refer to figures; those in **bold** to tables

Printed in the United States
by Baker & Taylor Publisher Services